*Understanding
Alzheimer's Disease*

Understanding Alzheimer's Disease

What It Is
How to Cope with It
Future Directions

*Alzheimer's Disease and
Related Disorders Association*

Edited by Miriam K. Aronson, Ed.D.
Foreword by Robert N. Butler, M.D.

Charles Scribner's Sons

NEW YORK

Charles Scribner's Sons
Macmillan Publishing Company
866 Third Avenue, New York, NY 10022
Collier Macmillan Canada, Inc.

This book is not intended as a substitute for the medical advice of physicians. The reader should regularly consult a physician in matters relating to his/her health care and particularly to any symptoms that may require diagnosis or medical attention.

Library of Congress Cataloging-in-Publication Data
Understanding Alzheimer's disease.

Bibliography: p.
Includes index.
1. Alzheimer's disease—Popular works.
I. Aronson, Miriam K.   II. Alzheimer's Disease and
Related Disorders Association. (Chicago, Ill.)
[DNLM: 1. Alzheimer's Disease—popular works.
WM 220 U55]
RC523.U53   1987   362.1'969792'00973   87-5037
ISBN 0-684-18475-3

Macmillan books are available at special discounts for bulk purchases for sales promotions, premiums, fund-raising, or educational use. For details, contact:

Special Sales Director
Macmillan Publishing Company
866 Third Avenue
New York, NY 10022

10 9 8 7 6 5 4 3
Designed by Nancy Sugihara
Printed in the United States of America

To the many millions of caring
people to whom dementia patients,
ADRDA, and society are indebted,
with the hope that in the future
the mechanism(s) underlying dementing
illness will be understood and the
ravages of it, therefore, unknown

Contents

PART II
How to Cope

Foreword

THE AGING OF AMERICA during this century has been a triumph of modern medicine and favorable economic conditions. There have been gains at both ends of the life cycle. Thanks to better prenatal, perinatal, and pediatric care and the development of vaccines and antibiotics, more people are able to survive into adulthood. Advances regarding management of infection and postponement or prevention of cardiovascular disease have helped more people survive into old age, and because of better management of chronic disease, people are surviving longer.

This increased survival is a double-edged sword, since many older, frailer individuals fall prey to some of the more age-related diseases such as dementia. In 1974, when I was writing *Why Survive? Being Old in America*,* I noticed the tendency to regard "senility" as inevitable. Fortunately, since that time there has been increasing awareness in both the

*Robert N. Butler, *Why Survive? Being Old in America* (New York: Harper & Row, 1975).

public sector and the scientific community that the predominant form of senility is, in fact, a disease or a collection of diseases labeled Alzheimer's. This recognition is a message of hope. No longer is Alzheimer's disease (AD) considered a natural consequence of advanced age; rather, it is a problem that can be subjected to scientific study just like any other disease, leaving us with the promise that it might be treatable and someday curable.

In the meantime, AD and other dementing illnesses remain a major robber of quality of life among older Americans, depriving some four million persons of the opportunity to function at their best and causing their loved ones heartbreak and grief. While great strides have been made in raising consciousness about this affliction and some success registered in attracting new research interest and dollars, the activity is not yet commensurate with the enormity of the problem. For those currently affected, the health-care system does not meet their increasing needs for care and management over several years. Finally, the potential for financial devastation looms large, since the systems of insurance, both public and private, are not geared to this devastating chronic illness.

Before 1974 there was a tendency to write off people who showed signs of senility, to regard them as untreatable and incurable. Since that time, and in no small measure as a result of the distinctive contribution of the Alzheimer's Disease and Related Disorders Association (ADRDA), it has become clear that much can be done to improve the lives of Alzheimer victims if patients and caregivers can maximize their coping abilities.

This book can help. It is geared toward caregivers and those health professionals who work with them, providing much-needed information about AD and related disorders in a general sense as well as in terms of specific, day-to-day management strategies. It provides state-of-the-art information regarding the dementias: how they are diagnosed, how they are managed, and what treatment strategies are available. Families can learn about the disease not as an abstract entity but in the context of how it impacts on their lives. The information is presented in straightforward language. Almost every chapter is freestanding, so that family members can read intermittently one chapter or one section at a time to answer their current questions or concerns. The book has an especially strong section on legal and financial issues, emphasizing the importance of advance planning to assure acceptable levels of care for the patient without pauperization of the family.

Pragmatic advice is provided regarding some of the most common symptoms exhibited by the patient: wandering, sleeplessness, agitation, changes in sexual behavior. Emphasis is placed on maintaining an optimal level of function in the patient.

The health of caregivers is also considered, and an effort is made throughout the book to address the considerable emotional wear and tear they experience, with advice on how to reduce stress. Caregivers are given practical information, too: what to tell the patient, how to get a diagnosis, what to look for in a support group, how to look for services, how to get through the placement process; and technical terms are defined and explained in glossaries that follow several of the chapters.

Since the publication of *Why Survive? Being Old in America*, some progress has been made. The National Institute on Aging was established, and through it a national initiative on AD was generated. Considerable, albeit insufficient, funding has been provided for research into the cause and cure of AD. We hope that in another decade or less the fear associated with survival into old age will be further reduced by definitive contributions to the understanding and treatment of the disease. Until that time, we're all fortunate to have ADRDA, the national voluntary health organization that is genuinely concerned about the plight of dementia victims and their families and that, in a few short years, has brought AD out of the closet—from a "silent epidemic" to almost a household word. ADRDA is an advocacy group that works for, among other things, more and better professional and public education about AD, research, and financial support for home care and other long-term services so that more of us will be able to have happier, more productive older years.

ROBERT N. BUTLER, M.D.

Acknowledgments

I WOULD LIKE TO ACKNOWLEDGE the enthusiasm and wisdom of the contributors, who helped to give this book a breadth and depth that will help satisfy the tremendous need to know of AD patients and their families.

My colleagues and friends provided invaluable review and insight. I would especially like to acknowledge Renee Pollack, Education Committee Chair, and Dr. Marrott Sinex, Public Policy Committee Chair, Richard Gelula, Associate Executive Director, Alzheimer's Disease and Related Disorders Association, and Jerome H. Stone, President, Alzheimer's Disease and Related Disorders Association. Drs. Leon Thal, of San Diego, Francois Boller, of Pittsburgh, and Howard Crystal, of New York, Robert Kruger, Esq., and Elaine S. Yatzkan, A.C.S.W., were especially helpful.

I applaud the efforts of Katherine Wild, M.A., and Paula Amerman, R.N., M.S., for critical review and invaluable editorial assistance. Janet Feroce tirelessly typed and assumed responsibility for manuscript preparation. Betsy Rapoport, our editor, was most helpful—and more important, patient.

Most of all, I express my gratitude to the courageous AD patients and their families and the hundreds of volunteer research subjects with whom I have worked over the years, who are a continuous source of inspiration and information.

MIRIAM K. ARONSON, ED.D.

PART I

Alzheimer's Disease and Related Disorders: Definitions, Diagnosis, and Treatment

CHAPTER ONE

Alzheimer's Disease and Related Disorders: An Overview

Peter Davies, Ph.D.

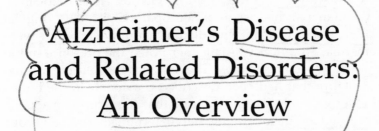

DEMENTIA IS A DETERIORATION in intellectual performance that always involves memory loss and is severe enough to interfere with work or social activities or both. There is almost always a loss of problem-solving ability and other aspects of abstract thinking, as well. Alzheimer's disease (AD) is the most common form of dementia.

For many years, the term "Alzheimer's disease" was used to denote what was thought to be a rare presenile dementia, that is, dementia in persons under age sixty-five. Several studies over the last few years clearly indicate that AD, in addition to being the major cause of dementia in persons under sixty-five, is the largest single cause of senile dementia, that is, dementia in persons over sixty-five, as well.

It has been estimated that about 15 percent of the U.S. population aged sixty-five and over, or 4.4 million persons, suffer from senile dementia. AD has an increasing incidence and prevalence with advancing age. While fewer than 1 percent of persons are affected at age sixty-five, this statistic

3

rises steeply to 20 percent of those aged eighty and older. AD is democratic, affecting adults regardless of gender, ethnic group, or socioeconomic circumstance.

AD was originally described in 1906 by Alois Alzheimer, a German psychiatrist and neuropathologist. His original patient was a woman who died at age fifty-six with severe dementia. At autopsy, Alzheimer noted the presence in the brain of two abnormalities. The first was the neuritic plaque, a structure that had been described previously in the brains of elderly people. We now know that the neuritic plaque is composed of degenerating nerve terminals and a fibrous material called amyloid surrounded by glial cells that bind nerve-cell tissue together. The second abnormality noted by Alzheimer was the neurofibrillary tangle, a structure within nerve cells that stained heavily with the then recently introduced silver stain. The presence of the neurofibrillary tangle within nerve cells had not been described before, and it was this abnormality that defined a new disease. It was unfortunate that the first patient in which this disease was discovered was so young: this led physicians of the period to think of AD as a presenile dementia. Because dementia in individuals aged sixty-five or younger is, in fact, quite rare, it was not perceived to be a major health problem. This belief held back research into AD.

We now know differently: AD and related dementias pose a threat not only to those persons who are afflicted but to their families, friends, and ultimately to our society. The threat is so great that AD has been called "the disease of the century" by Lewis Thomas, noted physician and author. Said former Health and Human Services Secretary Margaret Heckler in a 1984 report: "When we find a cure for Alzheimer's disease, we—as a people—will release and reap a now untapped harvest of wisdom, insight, and experience from millions of Americans in their golden years."

Why the renewed interest, and why now? There are two factors that have reawakened interest in AD in recent years.

The first is the growing realization that populations in developed nations are aging. Largely because of improvements in public health and living standards, an increasing proportion of the population lives to advanced ages. In the United States in 1980, about 11 percent of the population was sixty-five or older, but even more important, those persons who are eighty-five or older represent the fastest-growing age group in our population. It is anticipated that those over seventy-five, who are the most vulnerable to AD, will comprise at least half of those over sixty-five by the year 2000. Since those over seventy-five require greater amounts of health and social services, their unprecedented longevity will continue to raise crucial issues in terms of economic and social costs.

The second factor is the realization that AD is the largest cause of dementia. Surveys in the United States, Europe, and Japan have uncovered the fact that between 50 and 60 percent of patients dying with dementia have the pathological changes characteristic of AD: that is, they have neuritic plaques and neurofibrillary tangles in their brains. A further 20 percent of demented patients have plaques and tangles in addition to other pathological abnormalities such as strokes. Therefore, AD at least contributes to dementia in about 70 percent of demented patients aged sixty-five years or over. The remainder of patients are largely stroke victims (about 20 percent of the total) or suffer from any one of fifty or so conditions that can produce dementia. These include brain tumors, hypothyroidism, pernicious anemia, head injuries, reactions to drug treatment, certain infections of the brain, etc. Severe depression in the elderly is quite easy to mistake for dementia because of the patient's characteristic lack of responsiveness and apathy.

There are two points to be kept in mind. One, the majority of elderly persons who exhibit symptoms of dementia will turn out to have AD. Two, there are other causes of dementia symptoms that may be treatable. Thus, every person with these symptoms deserves a thorough medical investigation.

Symptoms

The symptoms of AD include gradual declines in memory, learning, attention, and judgment; disorientation in time and space; word-finding and communication difficulties; and changes in personality. These symptoms may be somewhat vague at first and mimic mental illness or stress-related problems. For example, an executive may not be managing as well as he once did, making bad decisions with increasing frequency and missing deadlines. Insidiously but inexorably, the changes become pronounced; the same executive who was responsible for the management of millions of dollars may become unable to add two numbers together. Similarly, a previously talented hostess may no longer be able to set a table. The personality of the patient may change markedly: an outgoing, vivacious person may become quiet and withdrawn; a gentle, caring partner may become aggressive and indifferent. Emotional symptoms, including depression, paranoia, and agitation, may occur intermittently. During the course of the illness, the patient's needs for care escalate. Of the four-plus million Americans with dementia, one-third are so impaired that they can no longer manage without assistance in the simplest daily routine activities of eating, dressing, grooming, and toileting.

Dementia affects at least 60 percent of nursing-home residents, and the cost of their nursing-home care runs into billions of dollars yearly. However, most persons with dementia reside at home, and most are cared for by family members. Because of the long-term burdens on them and the potential physical and emotional consequences, family members are recognized as the secondary victims of AD.

Perhaps the most important result of the current interest

in AD is the recognition of the importance of a good diagnosis. This is not a trivial matter, because at the moment there is no single diagnostic test for AD. A careful history, a mental-status test, and a comprehensive physical examination are essential. In addition, blood samples must be submitted to chemical analysis for various substances, including thyroid hormones and vitamin levels; spinal-fluid samples may be checked for the presence of abnormal cells or proteins; and computerized axial tomography (CT) scanning) can be used to determine whether there is evidence of strokes or tumors. Electroencephalography (EEG) may be used to check the brain's electrical activity. Psychological testing may be performed to identify strengths and weaknesses. A diagnosis of AD can be considered when other causes of dementia have been ruled out and the findings are consistent with AD. This diagnosis can be confirmed only by brain biopsy or at autopsy.

Treatment

Currently there is no established treatment for AD, although research in this area has grown dramatically in the last few years. The stimulus for this growth has come from neurochemical investigations of brains removed at autopsy from patients with AD. A breakthrough came in 1976, when three groups working in Great Britain uncovered evidence of a major deficiency in acetylcholine production in several regions of the brain. Acetylcholine is a chemical neurotransmitter used by a small proportion of nerve cells in the brain to transmit signals to other nerve cells. Because there was evidence from both human and animal experimentation that interference with acetylcholine transmission impairs memory function, it was tempting to speculate that at least some of the symptoms of AD were due to a deficiency of that neurotransmitter. More recent work tends to support this speculation. There are correlations between the extent of the problem with acetylcholine production and the degree of dementia assessed before death and with the number of neuritic plaques found at autopsy in the cerebral cortex. We now believe that the deficiency of acetylcholine results from the death of a small group of cells in an area deep in the brain, called the nucleus basalis of Meynert.

One of the most vexing questions at this time concerns the specificity of the deficit in acetylcholine production. We know of at least twenty compounds in the brain that seem to be used as transmitters of information between cells, and more are being identified every year. Is the production of all transmitters affected by AD, or is it just acetylcholine? Unfortunately, we cannot yet provide a complete answer to the question. Of eleven other transmitter substances investigated, the best that can be said is that the acetylcholine deficiency in Alzheimer patients seems to be the most consistent and dramatic. Some problems have been reported to occur in the nerve cells that use noradrenaline as their transmitter, but currently available information indicates that these are present in only a relatively small proportion of Alzheimer patients. The same may be true of nerve cells that use serotonin, somatostatin, or gamma-aminobutyric acid as their transmitter. Nerve cells that use vasopressin, vasoactive intestinal peptide, cholecystokinin octapeptide, thyrotropin-releasing factor, substance P, dopamine, or leutinizing hormone–releasing hormone as transmitters seem to be largely unaffected by AD except perhaps in the very late stages. The picture that seems to be emerging is one in which there is a dramatic loss of acetylcholine-producing cells in all Alzheimer patients, with a lesser and quite variable involvement of other nerve cells, especially in very severely affected, late-stage cases.

No widely effective treatment for the cognitive symptoms of AD is available. Even if a successful treatment for the acetylcholine deficiency that seems to cause the symptoms of AD could be found, it would not be the whole solution. We need to understand why the acetylcholine-producing cells die. What is it that has the ability to seemingly select these cells for destruction? Several theories have been advanced to explain the cause of the disease, but at this time the available evidence is so limited that we don't know which will be the definitive theory.

Searching for a Cause

A popular guess at the moment is that a viral infection causes the cell death. This has gained support because of work on a rare form of dementia called Creutzfeldt-Jakob (CJ) disease, which has been shown to be transmissible from people to a variety of animals, including monkeys. The transmission is usually accomplished by the injection of brain tissue from patients who died with CJ disease into the brains of animals. The transmission has characteristics such that the presence of an agent that can multiply in the animal brain is beyond doubt, but so far the nature of the agent is not clear. If it is a virus, then it is unusual, because it takes a very long period to cause disease (from one to five years in monkeys) and because conventional virus-detection methods do not give a hint to its presence.

The relevance of this work to AD is not yet clear. The pathology of the two diseases is very different. Numerous attempts to transmit AD to animals have not succeeded, and conventional virus-detection methods have failed to reveal any evidence for the presence of a virus. It is possible that a virus causes AD, but if one does, it must be even more unusual than that which causes CJ disease.

One of the major concerns to the relatives of patients with AD is the possibility that it is an inherited disorder. This seems to be true in only a very small percentage of cases. In a few families, however, there is evidence that the disease is an error in the genetic material that is passed down from generation to generation, with half of the offspring inheriting the error. However, for the vast majority of cases, the disease appears to occur as a random event, with only a very small increase in the risk of close relatives getting the disease. As mentioned earlier, about 15 percent of those over sixty-five are demented to some degree; if you have twenty-five relatives aged over sixty-five, on average four will suffer from dementia. By simple chance, this number could be as high as six or eight, without any genetic influence at all. Most of the genetic studies suggest that the close relatives of patients have a slightly greater risk of contracting AD. While there are several other possible causes of AD, including environmental factors and abnormalities in the immune-defense system, there is so little evidence in these areas that we can only guess at their possible significance. Genetic factors are discussed in more detail in chapter 3.

Related Disorders

The clinical symptoms of AD can be produced by a number of other conditions. Even after the most sophisticated clinical examination, about 10 percent of patients autopsied prove not to have the plaques and tangles characteristic of AD. Many diseases can produce Alzheimer-like symptoms, although only four or five occur frequently enough to be discussed here as related disorders.

MULTI-INFARCT DEMENTIA (MID)

There are some patients with a number of small strokes who appear to have clinical features similar to those of AD.

One form of a stroke occurs if part of the brain is suddenly deprived of its normal blood supply. This type of stroke can occur when a blood clot gets lodged in an artery within the brain and blocks the flow of blood past that blood clot. Another common stroke occurs if "hardening of the arteries" (atherosclerosis) becomes so severe in a particular brain artery that blood cannot flow past an area of severe narrowing. Twenty years ago, many physicians believed that the majority of cases of dementia were due to atherosclerosis of brain arteries. We know now that atherosclerosis of brain arteries is associated with dementia only when the atherosclerosis is also associated with multiple cerebral infarcts (strokes).

Most persons would recognize such common forms of stroke as when a person suddenly becomes unable to move his right or left side or becomes unable to speak. Very small strokes can also occur. Often these strokes are so tiny that no obvious clinical problems are associated with them. However, after a person suffers from several small strokes, the combined effects of these small strokes can sometimes be associated with dementia. Persons who have had several large strokes can also become demented.

Both of these types of dementia resulting from multiple cerebral strokes are called multi-infarct dementia (MID). Several features distinguish MID from AD. Patients with MID often (but not always) have a history of having had a stroke in the past, may have evidence of an old stroke on CT scan or MRI (magnetic resonance imaging) scan and may have focal signs (such as weakness of one side of their body) on neurological exam. Treatment of the underlying factors that may have contributed to the stroke, such as high blood pressure, may prevent further strokes and thereby prevent progression of dementia in some of these patients.

Many subjects have a combination of both multiple strokes and AD contributing to their dementia. These patients are said to have a "mixed" dementia.

BINSWANGER'S DISEASE

A very controversial cause of dementia is Binswanger's disease. This type of dementia is associated with severe changes in many of the arteries in the brain.

Binswanger's disease is a form of MID. Patients typically exhibit motor difficulty, especially dysarthria (difficulty articulating words) and dysphagia (difficulty swallowing). The disease evolves over several months, and is characterized by prolonged plateaus. The duration of the illness is long in comparison with other types of dementia. All reported cases of patients with Binswanger's have had hypertension. It was once felt that Binswanger's disease is exceedingly rare, but the incidence of Binswanger's disease is now being reinvestigated.

PARKINSON'S DISEASE

Patients with Parkinson's disease may also exhibit cognitive changes. Many Parkinsonian patients may seem "slow" in their thinking processes but if given enough time will demonstrate that they can think adequately. Some Parkinsonian patients may have relatively specific problems with their ability to remember where objects are arranged in space but have few other cognitive problems.

Parkinsonian patients may become depressed frequently, possibly because of neurotransmitter changes within their brains. Depression can make patients very apathetic and thus appear cognitively impaired. This kind of depression sometimes is helped with antidepressant medication.

Some investigators believe that some patients who have had Parkinson's disease for several years will also develop AD. Subjects with Parkinson's disease who also develop AD will gradually develop increasingly severe dementia superimposed on the problems with movement that are characteristic of Parkinson's disease. On the other hand, many patients with severe AD develop some of the features of Parkinson's disease such as very slow walking, stiffness, and difficulty getting in and out of chairs, although they may not experience tremor.

CREUTZFELDT-JACOB (CJ) DISEASE

CJ disease is extremely rare, occurring in about one per million people. Patients with CJ disease usually can be correctly diagnosed when they show characteristic changes in the electroencephalogram or a very rapid progression of symptoms. The course of the disease is usually rapid, rarely more than two years. As discussed, CJ seems to be caused by a viruslike agent, since it can be experimentally transmitted to animals. However, there is no evidence of person-to-person transmission, and the disease should not be considered contagious.

PICK'S DISEASE

Pick's disease can be very difficult to distinguish clinically from AD. Patients with Pick's disease often have marked behavioral symptoms such as social inappropriateness, loss of modesty, and disinhibited sexual behavior, while their memory is relatively mildly impaired. On CT scan or magnetic resonance imaging (MRI), they often have a very striking atrophy of the temporal cortex, more marked than is seen in AD. At autopsy, diagnosis is confirmed by the absence of plaques and tangles and the presence of "Pick bodies" in nerve cells. Perhaps fewer than 1 in 100 patients with AD proves to have Pick's disease. An even rarer cause of dementia is Pick-like cases, in which there is striking atrophy of the temporal lobe but no Pick bodies. Patients with the latter condition (which we call lobar atrophy) often have all of the classic symptoms of AD, but some do not seem to suffer as much memory loss as others.

HUNTINGTON'S DISEASE

Very rarely, patients with Huntington's disease are diagnosed as having AD. Huntington's disease is an inherited disorder that usually presents as a movement disorder, with the patients making frequent involuntary movements of all body parts. Psychiatric disturbance such as hallucinations, paranoia, and depression may be prominent early in the course. Dementia is usually found late in the course of the disease but can sometimes be the presenting symptom. Because movement disorders are rarely a feature of AD, the development of such symptoms would usually lead to a revision of the diagnosis.

It is perhaps appropriate to end this overview on an optimistic note. When all the figures are compiled, it is clear that the majority of the population will avoid this dreadful condition, whatever age group we are talking about. Even among people over eighty, four out of five will live their lives without any signs of dementia. The very dramatic progress research has made toward understanding AD offers some real hope that the next few years will see the development of a successful treatment for the symptoms of this condition. It seems clear now that AD is a specific disease, not an inevitable result of getting old. It is a disease that we should be able to beat if we are willing to put the necessary resources into research. It seems obvious that this must be done, because this is one disease that will become more and more common as advances in other areas of medicine allow increasing numbers of people to survive into the age of higher risk. It would indeed be a hollow victory if we prolong life without ensuring that the additional time can be enjoyed.

CHAPTER TWO

The Diagnosis of Alzheimer's Disease and Other Dementing Disorders

Howard A. Crystal, M.D.

THE EARLIEST SYMPTOM OF Alzheimer's disease (AD) is usually memory loss. Other symptoms include problems with learning, attention, judgment, and orientation; difficulty in finding the right word; and changes in personality and behavior.

Not all older patients with memory problems have AD. Memory impairment can result from more than fifty disorders, including the side effects of drugs, metabolic abnormalities, vitamin or hormonal deficiencies, and small "silent" strokes. Excessive anxiety or depression can also produce symptoms that simulate a memory disorder. This chapter reviews how physicians diagnose AD on the basis of history of the illness, physical and psychological examinations, and laboratory tests.

Some persons with memory problems will say that they don't remember things because "they're not important." This may be a cover-up. Distinguishing between "normal" age-related memory changes and early AD can be difficult. No single test will prove whether a person has AD or a related

15

dementing disorder. Evaluation should be obtained when memory and thinking deteriorate to the extent that a person either cannot function socially or work at his or her usual level.

Mr. S., an eminent real estate broker, was hospitalized for a prostate operation. While he was in the hospital, it was obvious to the physicians and nurses that he was very confused. His wife said he had been confused "for only a few weeks." She said that he could not have been confused for a long time, since he had been working as a broker until the week prior to his hospitalization. Because the consulting neurologist doubted this history, he asked for permission to interview the patient's secretary. The secretary said that her boss had been badly confused for three years. Junior members of his firm had been covering for him. The secretary would draw up the necessary forms and have her boss sign them in the appropriate places. In all likelihood, the broker's impairments had been present for several years.

Other changes in cognition that should always be evaluated include hallucinations, unusual or uncharacteristic agitation, getting lost, and changes in personality.

If worry about memory loss is a source of constant anxiety to either the affected individual or a member of his or her family, it is best to seek an evaluation. In such cases, the physician must *first* determine whether the patient, in fact, has a cognitive impairment.

Mr. D. was a forty-five-year-old executive who said that his mother "became senile" at the age of seventy-five. After forgetting to meet his wife for a noontime luncheon appointment, he became convinced that he was developing AD. Mr. D. was functioning at a very high level at work and was soon to be appointed his company's executive vice-president. Aside from this single missed appointment, he was functioning socially at his usual level. Detailed neuropsychological testing showed that Mr. D. was performing at a "gifted level." Review of his mother's history suggested that she had had several strokes and probably never had AD. Mr. D. was reassured that he didn't have AD. Yearly follow-up over the next ten years showed absolutely no evidence of decline.

Some people have a "fear of Alzheimer's disease." A person may forget a trivial appointment or an item his wife asked him to buy at the supermarket and become convinced that he has AD. Understandably, this fear is often worse in those persons who have family members with AD.

As in the case of Mr. D., if an individual is able to work with his usual competence, demonstrates no change in personality or social skills, and has normal mental-status testing and normal psychological tests, it is unlikely that one or two isolated memory lapses are early symptoms of AD. On the other hand, if a person is cognitively impaired, then the exact causes of the impairment must be identified.

The Importance of Diagnosis

"Dementia" is the medical term used to describe progressive impairment in memory and thinking so severe that it interferes with occupational or social function. AD is the most frequent cause of dementing illness and is responsible for 50–60 percent of these cases. The second most common cause of dementia is multiple small strokes. Often the cause of these strokes can be treated, making future strokes and further cognitive impairment less likely. Reversible causes of dementia include certain hormone imbalances and vitamin deficiencies, blood clots around the outside of the brain, seizures, the side effects of certain medications, excess swelling within the fluid-containing spaces of the brain (known as hydrocephalus), infections, certain psychiatric conditions (including depression), and some brain tumors. Unsuspected liver or kidney disease or high blood calcium levels sometimes cause symptoms similar to those of AD. Identifying a reversible cause of dementia may permit appropriate treatment so that the individual can return to his normal level of function.

Even if the diagnosis is AD—for which there is currently no therapy that reverses or slows its progression—early diagnosis may be valuable. It allows patients and families to plan appropriately for the future, including decisions regarding business activities, retirement, or changing residence. Appropriate investments can sometimes be made to provide funds that may be necessary for future care. Afflicted persons may choose to fulfill lifelong travel plans sooner than originally anticipated. In addition, the patient with an early diagnosis may be in the best position to take advantage of experimental drug-treatment trials that are available.

Making a Clinical Diagnosis

The diagnosis of AD is made on the basis of (1) establishing a history of illness compatible with this disorder, (2) documenting on a mental-status exam that the patient's memory deficits and other cognitive impairments are consistent with AD, (3) documenting on physical examination that other conditions such as Parkinson's disease or multiple strokes are not present, (4) performing laboratory tests to rule out disorders that can simulate AD, (5) obtaining a psychiatric evaluation, and (6) psychological testing.

HISTORY

The clinical course of AD is best characterized as a slow, progressive deterioration in memory and other intellectual functions, including language ability, ability to draw, and problem solving. The history of illness should be obtained from the patient (when possible) *as well as* from his or her spouse, children, and/or whoever else has relevant information, since the accuracy of the historical information is important in making a diagnosis. Some features of the history that should be reviewed are listed in table 2.1. Any evaluation that omits a substantial number of these ques-

Table 2.1

Features to Be Reviewed in the History

---

1. Duration and course of memory impairment. Did the problem start suddenly, or was it more gradual in onset?
2. Are there problems with language?
3. Are there problems with judgment?
4. Have there been changes in personality?
5. Is there evidence of depression, apathy, or agitation?
6. Specific evidence of decline
   a. When did the patient become unable to handle the checkbook?
   b. When did his or her housecleaning chores or cooking skills begin to deteriorate?
   c. Can he or she still work at his or her usual level?
   d. Can he or she still play games such as cards or do crossword puzzles?
   e. Does the patient get lost or confused in strange locales?
   f. Does he or she wash and dress himself or herself?
   g. How is his or her sleeping?
   h. Does he or she have changes in bladder or bowel habits?
   i. Has there been any change in his or her walking?
7. Is there a history of head trauma, strokes, seizures, or thyroid disease?
8. What are the patient's current medications, their reasons for use, and the patient's reactions to them?
9. Is there a history of previous psychiatric illnesses—such as depression?
10. Are there other medical illnesses or weight loss/gain?
11. Have there been relatives with similar changes in memory?
12. Does the patient complain of headaches or other pains?
13. Is the patient consistent in his behavior, or are there marked fluctuations in performance?

---

tions is too incomplete to be reliable. The physician obtaining the history will judge whether the history of the patient's illness is consistent with the usual pattern of AD.

MENTAL-STATUS EVALUATION

Mental status is determined by assessing the individual's ability to abstract, use symbols, and evaluate new experiences on the basis of past experience. There are several standardized mental-status tests in use. Simple items from two of those most commonly used are shown in table 2.2.

No single error on a mental-status test proves whether or not a patient has AD. It is the nature of the errors considered as a whole that is most important. Persons with limited schooling are, in general, less likely to know certain facts such as the dates of the world wars. No one would deny, however, that a history teacher who has no idea of the dates of World War II is impaired. On the other hand, a person for whom English is a second language, who has had limited formal education and has always worked at jobs that were relatively undemanding intellectually, can make several errors on the types of questions listed in table 2.2 and still not be diagnosed as having a dementing illness. Finally, the questions in table 2.2 may be too simple for some people. A physicist who is accustomed to solving difficult theoretical problems may answer all of the questions in table 2.2 without difficulty but may no longer be able to work at his profession. Therefore, the physician must consider the background and training of the individual to interpret the mental-status examination results.

GENERAL PHYSICAL EXAMINATION

The physician evaluates the patient's nutritional status, checks blood pressure and pulse, and searches for the presence of cardiac or respiratory disease, liver or kidney disease, or

Table 2.2

Samples of Questions Asked in Mental-Status Exams

---

1. What year is it now?
2. What month is it now?
3. What date is it now?
4. What is the day of the week?
5. Repeat a five-item test phrase (e.g., a name and an address) and then recall it several minutes later.
6. Give the name of the current president and immediately preceding president.
7. Give the dates of World Wars I and II.

SOURCE: Blessed, G., Tomlinson, B. E., and Roth, M. 1968. Association between quantitative measure of dementia and of senile change in the cerebral grey matter of elderly subjects. *Br. J. Psychiatry* 114:797–811.

1. Begin with 100 and count backward by 7.
2. Spell "world" backward.
3. Show a pencil and a watch and ask patient to name them.
4. Repeat the following: "No ifs, ands, or buts."
5. Follow a three-stage command: "Take a paper in your right hand, fold it in half, and put it on the floor."
6. Write a sentence.
7. Copy a design.

SOURCE: Folstein, M. F., Folstein, S., and McHugh, P. R. 1975.Mini-mental state: a practical method for grading the cognitive state of patients for the clinician. *J. Psychiatr. Res.* 12:189–98.

generalized atherosclerosis (sometimes called "hardening of the arteries").

NEUROLOGICAL EXAMINATION

A neurological exam is performed to look for evidence of previous strokes, Parkinson's disease, hydrocephalus, and other illnesses that can impair thinking. A neurological exam will include medical-history questions and a mental-status examination.

LABORATORY STUDIES

The physician will order a number of laboratory studies, including (1) various blood tests, (2) an electroencephalogram (EEG), and (3) a CT scan or MR scan to determine if other illnesses are present that can simulate AD.

Blood Tests Routine blood chemistries are obtained to measure blood calcium levels as well as kidney and liver function. High blood calcium levels or abnormal kidney or liver function can sometimes cause problems in thinking. A complete blood count (CBC) and sedimentation rate (ESR) are obtained because they can signal the presence of chronic infections or tumors that could cause cognitive problems.

The blood levels of vitamin B_{12} and folic acid are measured because a very low level of these vitamins is sometimes associated with dementia. Correction of the deficiencies may improve or even reverse the dementia.

Thyroid function is measured because very low or very high amounts of thyroid hormone can be associated with confusion or slowing of brain function similar to dementia. Correcting the thyroid abnormality may eliminate the patient's confusion.

A blood test for venereal disease should be performed because prolonged (probably greater than twenty years) syphilitic infection can sometimes cause dementia. Around 1900, this form of dementia was very common, but since the discovery of penicillin, it has become rare.

Electroencephalogram (EEG) An EEG (or electroencephalogram) is a record of the brain's electrical activity. There are two reasons for obtaining an EEG. First, persons with epilepsy can have subtle seizures that are not readily noticed by family members. Patients who suffer from these untreated seizures can so often be confused that they appear demented. Second, patients with AD should have normal or "diffusely slow" EEG patterns. If a patient appears very demented but has a perfectly normal EEG, then it is possible that a severe psychiatric illness is responsible for some or all of his problems.

The CT Scan CT scanning (computerized axial tomography) is an imaging technique whereby X rays are passed through the body part under examination and changes in the X-ray beams are analyzed by a computer. The purpose of the CT scan of the brain in evaluating patients with memory changes is to look for problems other than AD that can cause memory impairment. Some of these other causes include brain tumors, strokes, blood clots, and hydrocephalus.

CT scans may also reveal normal changes in the brain. The normal brain shrinks a little with aging, a condition called atrophy. Therefore, the brain of a normal seventy-year-old is likely to be a little smaller than the brain of a twenty-year-old. On average, seventy-year-old Alzheimer patients will have more brain atrophy visible on a CT scan than normal seventy-year-olds. However, this finding alone is not diagnostic of AD.

Other Brain-Imaging Techniques An MRI (magnetic resonance imaging) scan (also called NMR scan) is a brain-imaging technique that is similar in some ways to CT scanning.

In MRI scanning, magnetic beams rather than X rays are used for imaging.

The relative merits of both kinds of scans are still being evaluated; nonetheless, there are instances in which ambiguities raised by the findings on a CT scan suggest the need for a more detailed picture via an MRI scan. In general, either a CT scan or an MRI scan should be part of a dementia evaluation.

PET Scanning The PET scan (positron emission tomography) is an experimental technique whereby a short-lived radioisotope is injected into the vein or artery of the patient and brain images are taken with a device somewhat similar to a CT scan. PET scans differ from either CT scans or MRI scans in that the PET scans measure the chemical activity (metabolism) of the brain. The PET scans of many patients with AD will show decreased metabolism in specific regions of their brains; however, the PET scan is not able to give a specific diagnosis of AD because similar patterns of decreased brain metabolism can be caused by a number of illnesses. The PET scan is a powerful research tool but is not an accepted part of the routine evaluation of a patient suspected of having AD because it is experimental and not widely available.

Spinal Tap Some physicians perform a spinal tap (lumbar puncture) as a routine part of a dementia evaluation. Lumbar punctures may help to identify infections or malignancies that may be responsible for cognitive changes. Further, researchers are currently searching for a substance in spinal fluid unique to AD. If this is discovered, then a spinal tap may be an important diagnostic tool for AD.

PSYCHIATRIC EVALUATION

Psychiatric evaluation is sometimes necessary to rule out the presence of illnesses such as depression. A severely depressed older person may suffer from memory loss that may mimic dementia. It is important that loss of memory due to depression be diagnosed, since this condition is potentially curable with the proper medications and other therapies. Additionally, depression can affect persons with dementia, especially earlier in the course of the illness.

PSYCHOLOGICAL TESTING

A battery of psychological tests may be needed to determine subtle changes in a patient's cognitive functioning. The psychologist administers tests to evaluate various elements of brain function, including memory, language, and constructional abilities. These tests are "normalized," so that data are available to show how normal patients of the same age and educational background perform. They are especially helpful in evaluating atypical cases. Some patients whose baseline intelligence was extremely high may do very well on routine measures used for mental-status evaluation, yet clearly are declining in their ability to function. Neuropsychological testing can be helpful in these patients as well as in tracking the progression of a dementing illness.

Making a Diagnosis

If all of the parts of the evaluation are consistent with AD, the physician will conclude that AD is the most likely clinical diagnosis. In circumstances in which all features seem to fit the usual pattern of AD, this clinical diagnosis is correct 80–90 percent of the time.

Other Dementing Illnesses

Vascular dementia, or multi-infarct dementia (MID), the second most common cause of dementia, is due to a loss of brain tissue. This is the result of either a series of small, often imperceptible strokes or, occasionally, large strokes. It occurs most commonly in patients with untreated hypertension or diabetes but can also follow other events, such as cardiac arrest, carbon-monoxide poisoning, or shock. MID can occur together with AD; in fact, half of the patients with this condition have both small strokes and AD. Together the combined and pure multi-infarct dementias comprise about 35 percent of all patients with dementia. The onset of MID is usually sudden, and intellectual decline occurs in a more abrupt, "stepwise" fashion than in AD. The workup, or diagnostic assessment, for MID is similar to that for AD. Certain neurological signs and symptoms, such as weakness of an arm or leg, are more common in MID than in AD.

Pick's disease is a much rarer cause of dementia than AD. Many scientists think it is impossible to distinguish between Alzheimer's disease and Pick's disease on the basis of clinical history and neurological and psychiatric examination, and believe that Pick's disease can be accurately diagnosed only by brain biopsy or at autopsy. Other experts believe that subjects whose clinical picture is dominated by social and sexual inappropriateness and the tendency to become very oral when their memory is relatively intact are more likely to have Pick's disease than AD. Unfortunately, there is, as yet, no treatment that stabilizes or cures Pick's disease, and its late course is indistinguishable from that of AD.

Some patients with Parkinson's disease also become demented. Patients who develop Parkinson's disease in their seventies and eighties are particularly likely to become demented as their disease progresses. Dementia appears to be especially common in Parkinsonian patients whose major problem is slowness of movement (bradykinesia) and stiffness rather than tremor. Impairment in thinking in Parkinsonian patients may be caused by three different kinds of disorders. First, late in the course of their illness, many patients with Parkinson's disease also develop Alzheimer's disease. Second, some patients with Parkinson's disease develop a non-Alzheimer's dementia characterized mainly by poor memory and slowness of thinking. Third, many patients are very likely to become depressed, in part because of the brain changes caused by the disease. Treatment with medication may improve the depression associated with Parkinson's disease.

Brain tumors are another important cause of dementia. Patients whose dementia is due to brain tumors usually present with a somewhat different history and neurological exam than patients with AD. Nonetheless, sometimes the clinical history of patients with brain tumors can be very similar to that of patients with AD. Brain tumors can usually be easily diagnosed by CT or MRI scanning. Since nearly all brain tumors are treatable, and some are curable, it is important to be certain that brain tumors are not the underlying cause of a patient's dementia.

Getting a Diagnostic Assessment (Workup)

The diagnostic workup may be initiated by the family physician, an internist, a geriatrician, a neurologist, or a psychiatrist, each of whom may consult with the others. In any event, the diagnosing physician will review the results of examinations, laboratory studies, and other consultations to arrive at a diagnosis. An important part of the diagnostic process is educating the patient's family about the likely course of AD and what its implications will be for them as a family. AD is a complicated illness that requires attention not only from physicians but also from professionals of different disciplines, such as law, social work, nursing, counseling, and physical therapy. It's important that the family choose one professional to coordinate the patient's complete care. This coordination may be handled by the family physician or by another health professional in collaboration with the primary physician.

Ascertaining the Diagnosis

Many cases that eventually prove to be AD are not typical at the outset. Initially, some patients may only have memory impairment and no problem naming relatively obscure items or copying complex figures. Other patients may have intact memory but more marked problems naming objects and writing. Only when such patients are followed over a course of time—sometimes for several years—does the mental-status exam reflect that of most patients with AD. Unfortunately, persons with these "atypical" clinical histories may have a delayed diagnosis, with their families left to cope with the anxiety of diagnostic uncertainty.

As of this writing, the only way to be one hundred percent certain of the diagnosis of AD is to examine brain tissue under a microscope, by biopsy during life or autopsy after death. A brain biopsy is a surgical procedure whereby the patient is given a local anesthetic and a small piece of the brain is removed for examination under the microscope. If this specimen shows the characteristic microscopic changes of AD—large numbers of neurofibrillary tangles and senile plaques (fig. 2.1)—then the diagnosis is certain. Since a brain biopsy, like any surgical procedure, is associated with a small risk of infection or hemorrhage, it is almost never performed when the clinical diagnosis of AD appears likely.

After a patient dies, sections of the brain can be examined microscopically to determine whether the clinical diagnosis of AD was correct. Research scientists emphasize the continuing need for autopsy examinations of the brains of Alzheimer patients not only to confirm the diagnosis but to provide tissue for research into the causes of this disease.

Role of Repeat Evaluations

Without a specific test for AD, the clinical diagnosis can be difficult, especially very early in the course of the illness.

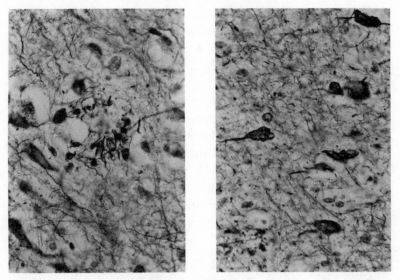

Figure 2.1. Senile plaques and neurofibrillary tangles are the pathologic hallmarks of Alzheimer's disease. **Right:** *A senile plaque. At the center of the plaque is a core of amyloid surrounded by degenerating nerve fibers (neurites).* **Left:** *Several cell bodies of nerve cells that contain neurofibrillary tangles.*

Even after a thorough evaluation of a person suspected of having AD, a physician may still be unable to make a diagnosis with any certainty.

> Mr. M. had very mild problems in thinking, and the family's local neurologist said that he didn't think Mr. M. had AD but that he couldn't be sure. Dissatisfied with the uncertainty, the family sought an opinion from a neurologist at a major medical center who was an "expert" on AD. After reviewing the patient's history and previous laboratory tests, doing a neurological exam, and obtaining a three-hour neuropsychological test battery, the consulting neurologist also wasn't certain whether Mr. M.'s cognitive problems were due to very early AD. The M. family was even more frustrated when they were told of this uncertainty. The consulting neurologist suggested that the patient return in six months for follow-up. At that time, although his cognitive deficits still remained quite mild, it was clear that

he was significantly worse than six months earlier. When examined a third time, a year after his initial evaluation, Mr. M. still showed relatively subtle problems, but it had become evident that the impairment was progressing. At that time, the family was told that Mr. M. had probable AD. Eight years later, the clinical diagnosis was confirmed upon autopsy.

In cases such as Mr. M., repeat evaluations at six-month or yearly intervals can be helpful. If no significant change occurs over this period of time, the diagnosis of AD becomes considerably less likely. On the other hand, if significant change does occur, even if a patient's deficits remain fairly mild, AD becomes a more likely diagnosis.

What to Tell the Patient

A question often asked by family members is "What do I tell the patient?" Some people are comfortable being candid and informing the patient that he or she has AD; others are no doubt reluctant. Most experts agree that in most cases it is in the best interests of both the patient and the family that the mildly impaired patient be told that he or she has AD. First, it prevents communication barriers between the patient and the family. Second, it gives the patient an explanation for his or her symptoms and reassurance that he or she is not "crazy." Third, and probably most important, it permits the mildly impaired patient to participate in planning his or her life.

Perspective and Summary

Around 1850, over half of the patients in mental institutions had general paresis of the insane—a dementing illness with psychotic features caused by syphilis. At that time, the cause of general paresis was as unknown as the cause of AD is today. A rapid understanding of the cause of general paresis came about with the discovery of the bacteria that causes syphilis in the brains of paretic patients. With the introduction of sulfa drugs and penicillin, general paresis has become virtually extinct. The history of general paresis is important because it gives perspective to the search for the discovery of the cause of and cure for AD. One hundred years ago, general paresis may have seemed so mysterious and complex a disease that it would never be understood. Discoveries that in retrospect seem simple but in their day were of profound significance led to a rapid unraveling of its mysteries. There is every reason to believe that in this era one or two equally profound discoveries will lead to an understanding of, and eventually a cure for, AD.

In summary, although there is, as yet, no one single test to prove whether a person has AD, a comprehensive evaluation results in a correct clinical diagnosis in 80–90 percent of cases. Obtaining a diagnosis is important not only because reversible conditions may be discovered and corrected in the process but also because patients and their families can plan appropriately. Every person with symptoms of intellectual and functional deterioration should receive a complete diagnostic evaluation.

Glossary

autopsy a procedure performed after death in which the body or specific parts of the body are closely examined to determine the cause of death. In order to diagnose AD, sections of the brain are examined microscopically to determine if the characteristic plaques and tangles are present.

biopsy a surgical procedure in which the patient is given an anesthetic and a small piece of brain tissue is removed and examined microscopically.

cognitive functions a broad term used to describe the quality of "knowing," which includes the ability to reason, judge, conceive, recognize, perceive, and imagine.

dementia the decline of memory and other intellectual functions from a person's previous level of function. Dementia may be caused by a number of diseases, the most common of which is AD. Multi-infarct dementia (MID) is caused by loss of brain tissue due to a series of small, often imperceptible strokes.

electroencephalogram (EEG) a record of the brain's electrical activity. It is obtained by attaching electrodes with paste to the skin of the head. A recording is then made while the patient quietly relaxes.

imaging techniques techniques such as X rays used to visualize body parts such as the brain. Some imaging techniques such as CT scans use X-ray beams, while others use magnetic beams (MRI or NMR scan) or radioisotopes (PET scan).

lumbar puncture also called an "LP" or "spinal tap." A lumbar puncture is a procedure by which spinal fluid is obtained for laboratory examination. An LP is a relatively safe procedure and is an important diagnostic tool if infection or malignancy is suspected.

References

Heston, L. L., and White, J. A. 1983. *Dementia: a practical guide to Alzheimer's disease and related illnesses*. New York: W. H. Freeman & Co., chap. 4, pp. 37–49. (Available through ADRDA)

Katzman, R. Fall 1982. The complex problem of diagnosis. *Generations* (Journal of the Western Gerontological Society) 7:8–10.

Khachaturian, Z. S. 1985. Diagnosis of Alzheimer's disease. *Arch. Neurol.* 42:1097–1105.

Mace, N. L., and Rabins, P. V. 1981. *The 36-hour day: a family guide to caring for persons with Alzheimer's disease, related dementing illnesses, and memory loss in later life.* Baltimore, Md.: The Johns Hopkins Univ. Press. (Available through ADRDA)

McKhann, G. et al. 1984. Clinical diagnosis of Alzheimer's disease. Report of the NINCDS–ADRDA Work Group under the auspices of the Department of Health and Human Services Task Force on Alzheimer's disease. *Neurology* 34:939–44. (Available through ADRDA)

CHAPTER THREE

Alzheimer's Disease: Possible Evidence for Genetic Causes

John C. S. Breitner, M.D., M.P.H.

THE CAUSE OF ALZHEIMER'S disease (AD) remains unknown. New information suggests several specific chemical and structural changes in the body that may be responsible for the symptoms of AD patients. To date, however, it is not known why some people develop these changes while others are spared.

One promising approach to this question is the study of the distribution of disease in populations. Such epidemiological studies may seek specific associations of the disease in question with one or more particular circumstances (risk factors) found only among affected individuals. Historically, such factors have been discovered at a time when the nature of their link to disease was not understood. Occasionally they offer clues to the ultimate causation of disease, which becomes fully apparent only on subsequent examination. Thus, in 1911, Goldberger found an association between the niacin-deficiency syndrome known as pellagra and an institutional diet. Only much later was the dietary deficiency understood to be specifically in the B-vitamin complex, and later still, a specific deficit in nicotinic acid. The exact mechanism by which nicotinic-acid deficiency causes destruction of specific structures in the nervous system is still under investigation.

Several studies in the present decade have examined possible risk factors for AD. To date, however, only three factors have been confirmed by more than one investigation. The two that are clearly established are age and genetic background. (The third, history of head injury, requires further investigation before it can be assigned a definite role.) The purpose of this chapter is to examine the evidence regarding genetic factors in the causation of AD. Because AD is found mainly in old age, unlike many well-known genetic disorders, the possible influence of heredity must be examined in terms of a predisposition to disease that may become evident only in old age.

Importance of Age in Genetic Studies

It is well known that the risk of AD increases dramatically with age. The rate of appearance of new cases, or incidence, accelerates markedly after age seventy-five and may reach 2 percent per year in the early ninth decade.* This strong association of AD with advanced age no doubt led in the past to the misconception that "senility" is a natural consequence of old age. While this view has been clearly disproved, it is true that the age of most probable onset of AD is also a time when the death rate (mortality) from all causes is extremely high. Therefore, much of any genetic predisposition may remain hidden among individuals who might

---

*Some evidence suggests that the incidence rate may begin to *decline* after about age eighty-five, but the data are not yet conclusive.

otherwise be destined to develop AD but who die first from another illness. This phenomenon poses problems for genetic analyses of AD, since the genetic makeup (genotype) of predisposed individuals is not always reflected in the actual appearance (phenotype) of the disease. The techniques required to deal with this problem will be introduced in the discussion of different kinds of genetic studies below.

Genetic Factors—the Evidence to Date

Numerous studies since the beginning of this century have demonstrated conclusively that the risk of AD is increased among those who have it in their family. One widely quoted estimate notes that the overall risk of AD-like illness is about fourfold greater among those with an affected first-degree relative (i.e., parent, sibling, or offspring) than in age-matched individuals with no affected first-degree relative. At age sixty-five this increased risk has little practical significance because the risk of AD at this age is extremely small. By age eighty, however, the risk to first-degree relatives is approximately 25 percent, as contrasted with 6 percent in the general population. This risk may suggest a genetic predisposition to AD in certain families, a suggestion that has been followed up by three different lines of inquiry: pedigrees, studies of relatives of AD patients, and the relation of AD to Down's syndrome.

PEDIGREES

Beginning in the 1930s, the medical literature contains numerous reports of isolated families in which AD is strikingly common. The largest and most completely studied pedigree (or family tree) showing the distribution of disease in one such family is reproduced in figure 3.1. Several features of

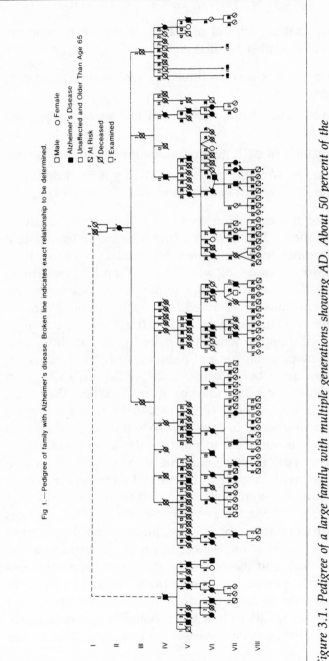

Fig 1.—Pedigree of family with Alzheimer's disease. Broken line indicates exact relationship to be determined.

☐ Male   ○ Female

■ Alzheimer's Disease

☐ Unaffected and Older Than Age 65

◪ At Risk

⊘ Deceased

◻ Examined

Figure 3.1. Pedigree of a large family with multiple generations showing AD. About 50 percent of the offspring of each affected individual eventually develop AD. Lack of disease in the youngest generations demonstrates the age-dependent nature of AD—those potentially at risk are too young to have expressed the disease. Approximately equal proportions of males and females are affected. The pattern is typical of that seen in diseases caused by the inheritance of an autosomal-dominant gene. (From L. E. Nee et al., A Family with Histologically Confirmed Alzheimer's Disease.)

this family that are typical of the more than fifty reported pedigrees of so-called familial AD:

1. The disease is seen in three or more successive generations.
2. Approximately equal numbers of males and females are affected.
3. About half of each generation eventually develop AD.
4. Owing presumably to their relative youth, individuals in the most recent generations show no disease.

Except for the last point, this pedigree is typical of those found in genetic disorders in which disease is transmitted by an autosomal-dominant genetic mechanism. Humans have forty-six chromosomes of which two (X and Y) determine sex, and forty-four, called autosomes, exist in twenty-two pairs (one chromosome derived from each parent at conception). Since humans have two of each autosome, one may ask what will happen when the paired genes at the particular locus or position on a chromosome differ. One gene, for example, may be defective and predispose to a given disease, while the other may be normal. When the genes differ in this way, an individual is said to be heterozygous at the particular locus in question. When a single dose of a harmful gene is sufficient to produce the known manifestations (phenotype) of that gene, the harmful gene is said to be dominant with respect to its normal counterpart. Examples of autosomal-dominant genetic diseases are Huntington's disease and Marfan's syndrome. Because the chances of any individual receiving the dominant harmful gene from his or her affected (usually heterozygous) parent are about fifty-fifty, about half the offspring of a given union containing an affected parent will receive the harmful gene and (ultimately) should develop the disease. Upon mating of such affected offspring, about half the succeeding generation will again show the specific disease, and so on. Because the chance inheritance of one or another autosome (with or without the harmful gene) is independent of the sex chromosomes, the disease is seen with roughly equal frequency among males and females.

Pedigrees such as that of figure 3.1 have been taken as evidence that AD can occur in a form in which its ultimate causation is hereditary and attributable to a predisposing autosomal-dominant gene. However, while AD is common, AD occurring with the frequency shown in figure 3.1 is extremely rare. Therefore, the lesson of the familial AD pedigrees is not that AD is generally transmitted via genetic mechanisms but rather that it *can* be so transmitted.

STUDIES OF RELATIVES

The major distinction between the disease in the familial AD pedigrees and its more typical counterpart is age at onset. Recall that the most probable age for expression of AD is in the seventies or even later. Almost invariably, however, the disease reported in the pedigrees begins in the forties and fifties. This is an age to which most individuals will survive. Thus, most individuals with the presumptive "familial AD" genotype will eventually show their predisposition to the illness. Such a finding would not be expected if a similar pattern of inheritability predisposed to the usual form of late-onset AD. Instead, many individuals with the presumptive AD genotype would then die of other causes before their disease was evident. The degree of actual manifestation of the presumptive gene would then depend on its characteristic age of expression and on the survival of the population.

The late age of onset of AD and the possibility of death from other illnesses make the study of these patients and their relatives difficult. These problems, however, can be bypassed to some extent, by the study of a pool of large numbers of relatives of many individual cases of AD and the application of biostatistical methods. Individuals diagnosed with AD are called index cases, or probands, while their relatives are referred to as proband relatives. If one can assemble 100 such probands and then take careful family histories from each, one can then study a population of several hundred first-degree relatives at risk. Many of these relatives (particularly parents) will be deceased, while others (especially offspring) will not yet have lived out their life span (and hence their entire period of risk for AD). What we can know about each is (1) his relation to the proband, (2) his age at last point of observation (whether age at death or current age), (3) whether he is affected with an AD-like dementing illness, and (4) if so, at what age the illness began.

This information is sufficient to construct a statistical model to analyze the age-specific risk of AD in the pooled proband relatives. In essence, one subdivides the population at risk into small groups on the basis of their age at last observation. Naturally, the size of these groups will diminish at the older age ranges, but if one starts with a large enough population at risk, even the oldest age ranges (say, eighty-six to ninety years) will be of sufficient size to allow meaningful analysis.

Provided the starting population is large enough, such risks can be studied throughout a theoretical human life span of ninety years or more. If the autosomal-dominant inheritance suggested by the reported familial AD pedigrees were also operative in late-onset AD, one would then expect that the cumulative incidence of AD, as estimated by these methods, would eventually reach 50 percent by some (perhaps very late) age. If, however, the initial group of index cases were heterogeneous in origin, containing both genetically transmitted cases and other, similar appearing but noninheritable cases, then the risks among their relatives would be correspondingly reduced.

Four groups of investigators have recently studied the risks of AD in proband families. The first and best known of these studies was conducted by Heston and colleagues (1981). They investigated familial risks for 125 individuals who had died in Minnesota state hospitals and had received an autopsy diagnosis of AD. (Autopsy diagnosis is generally considered definitive in AD,* and is essential for accurate retrospective studies.) The major findings of this study are as follows:

1. There were marked differences in familial risk in early-onset versus late-onset probands.

2. In early-onset disease (particularly where there was one affected relative) the risk to other first-degree family members increased with age and approached 50 percent by age ninety.

3. In all of twenty-five families in which a secondary case (a proband relative) had died and come to autopsy, the neuropathological diagnosis (based on observed structural and functional changes of the nervous system at autopsy) of the relative was identical to that of the proband.

4. The age of onset of the disease was significantly similar in family members.

5. Secondary cases tended to appear at ages considerably older than the index or proband cases.

When probands of all ages were considered jointly, the cumulative morbidity risk among their relatives reached 22 percent by age eighty-five. While the risk in early-onset proband families was far higher, that among families of the oldest probands scarcely exceeded risks found in control populations. Thus, these results do not support a simple interpretation that autosomal-dominant inheritance ac-

---

*It should be noted, however, that an *ante mortem* (before death) diagnosis of AD, when obtained by the use of standardized methods and the application of modern research diagnostic criteria, appears to yield greater than 90 percent diagnostic accuracy in most recent evaluations.

counts for familial risks in typical AD. While genetic factors may be operative, they appear from these studies to be more important in early-onset disease.

A different approach was used at Duke by Heyman and colleagues, who studied the families of sixty-eight AD cases diagnosed by clinical methods, all with onset of the illness before age seventy. Diagnostic criteria were similar to the newly proposed NINCDS/ADRDA standards (those defined by the National Institute of Neurological, Communicative Diseases and Stroke and the Alzheimer's Disease and Related Disorders Association) (McKhann et al., 1984), but the majority of probands showed only mild to moderate disease. Family studies showed greater age-specific incidence (cumulative incidence of 14 percent by age seventy-five) of AD among relatives than had been found in any previous investigation. Heston's finding of greater familial risk in early-onset cases was not replicated; however, the maximum age at onset of seventy years may have precluded a meaningful comparison. (Heston's early-onset cases had onset before sixty-five; the late-onset cases, mostly much later.)

Because of concerns about data reliability, Heyman et al. did not calculate familial risks in relatives over age seventy-five. This conservative practice may have resulted in loss of some potentially valuable data on older relatives. Still, these workers found dramatic differences in familial risks among relatives of AD probands as contrasted with relatives of spouse controls. It is noteworthy that the age-specific incidence (through age seventy-five) in this series equals or exceeds that in two studies (discussed below), which have been interpreted as suggesting dominant genetic disease in all AD probands.

A third study was reported by Breitner and Folstein (1984) from Johns Hopkins. These authors screened thirty-five hundred Baltimore nursing-home patients for AD using crude but standardized criteria. They found seventy-eight eligible subjects, of whom sixty-two (all white females) completed the study. A sample of thirty-three age- and sex-matched nursing-home controls was ascertained simultaneously. The probands were categorized by presence of the typical middle-stage AD symptoms, that is, aphasia (difficulties in language or speech) or apraxia (loss of ability to coordinate and execute learned motor tasks such as ability to comb one's hair, cut one's food, etc.): forty-two had developed such symptoms; eight had not but had been ill less than four years (hence, were thought likely still to develop them); and twelve had been ill over four years but were neither aphasic nor apractic. Family study then revealed a marked difference in AD risks among siblings and offspring of aphasic/apractic probands versus those patients lacking these symptoms. No secondary cases were observed among the fifty-six relatives of the latter group, while relatives of aphasic/apractic probands showed cumulative risks of AD exceeding 50 percent by age ninety. Nondemented nursing-home control relatives experienced a lifetime risk of 8 percent, which did not differ significantly from the risk observed among the proband's spouses. The observed lifetime incidence figures are consistent with the hypothesis that the aphasic/apractic probands had an autosomal-dominant genetic disorder. Since 78 percent of the proband sample had aphasia/apraxia, the authors suggested that a majority of AD-like illnesses might be genetically determined.

The Baltimore findings have been replicated in another series of clinically ascertained cases (Mohs et al., 1987). Like Heyman's, these fifty subjects were mainly ambulatory volunteers for clinical studies of AD. It is noteworthy that these cases were not originally ascertained for genetic studies. Thus, it is unlikely that the cases came forward out of concern about familial risk—an important potential source of bias in family studies of clinical populations. The NINCDS/ADRDA diagnostic criteria were employed, with the sole additional requirement that subjects must have shown a definite progression of severity in their symptoms over a one-year

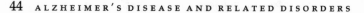

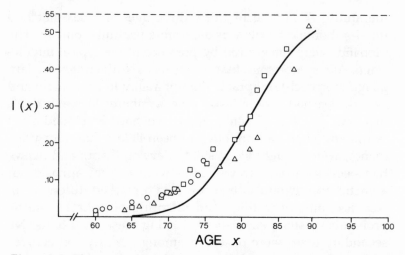

Figure 3.2. This composite figure shows cumulative incidence [I(x)] of AD in three studies (□ Mohs et al., 1987; △ Breitner and Folstein, 1984; ○ Heyman et al., 1983). The curve, which may be taken as broadly representative of risks as reported in recent studies, may be useful in future quantitative studies of the genetics of AD.

period. Age-matched (mainly spouse) controls were also investigated. As in the previous study, the estimated cumulative risk by age ninety for AD relatives was approximately 50 percent, while that for control relatives was much lower.

The last three studies combined appear to offer a coherent view of familial risks in AD, as suggested by figure 3.2. Each of these studies used clinical diagnoses of AD, obtained by application of structured diagnostic methods and criteria aimed at obtaining the purest possible diagnostic grouping obtainable without autopsy. The figure shows a curve that may be taken as a broadly applicable description of the risk of AD in such proband families. This curve of risk versus age is suggestive, but far from conclusive, of a view that AD as defined by careful clinical methods may be transmitted by the specific genetic mechanism of autosomal-dominant inheritance. The contrast between these results and Heston's is difficult to explain but may be due in part to the relatively common occurrence of senile plaques and neurofibrillary tangles in the brains of nondemented aged individuals (Tomlinson, 1982).

RELATION TO DOWN'S SYNDROME

Additional evidence linking AD to genetic factors is found in its relationship to Down's syndrome (DS), a known genetic disorder attributable to excess quantities of genetic material on human chromosome 21 (which results in a form of mental retardation sometimes called "mongolism"). This relationship is expressed in two different ways: there is increased prevalence of DS in AD proband families; and an AD-like neuropathological condition appears to develop invariably as DS patients approach the end of their usual life span of forty to fifty years. While it is not clear that these aging DS patients develop a clinical picture resembling AD, the neuropathological features include specific neural-tract changes and neurochemical abnormalities found in AD. Very recently, important new evidence has demonstrated an important role in AD for genes on chromosome 21. A DNA sequence polymorphism located in the long arm of this chromosome has now been tentatively linked (see following section) to a predisposition to AD in several families showing regular occurrence of early-onset disease. And another important gene with possible causal significance for AD has been identified in the same general region of this chromosome. The latter gene codes for the protein beta-amyloid, which is found in heavy deposits in the plaques that are an important characteristic of the neuropathology of AD. While the exact meaning of these findings remains unclear, they offer additional evidence that genetic factors play an important role in the biological changes that characterize the disease process in at least some cases of AD.

Twin Studies—Potential for Future Studies

To date, the problem of the late onset of AD has prevented the useful application of one of the most powerful, traditional methods of investigation in clinical genetics—twin studies.

Twin studies are particularly useful in distinguishing genetic from environmental influences. Since both fraternal and identical twins usually share a common environment, any difference in their potential for developing the disease is generally attributable to the differing degrees to which they share genetic material. Identical twins in which both members of the pair developed AD at similar ages have been reported, but identical twins with only one member affected have also been described. The largest reported twin study (Kallmann and Sander, 1949) found concordance rates (both having AD) of 42.8 percent in identical twins. Like all such studies, however, this one was troubled by the possibility that unaffected members of discordant pairs (one member with the disease, one without) may later develop AD. For instance, one study reported an identical twin pair in which onset of AD occurred in both, but at ages differing by fifteen years. Thus, until large-scale twin studies of AD are undertaken, the implications of these findings in AD will remain uncertain.

Conclusions

A variety of methodological problems have prevented the satisfactory analysis of genetic mechanisms as an explanation for the observed familial clustering in AD. Several recent advances have yielded new evidence suggesting ever more strongly that genetic factors may be powerful determinants of AD. With refinement in diagnostic procedures and new methods of family study, a few studies now suggest that autosomal-dominant inheritance may operate in large numbers of AD cases. The methods that could be used to confirm this hypothesis are still inadequate to the special problems posed by the late expression and difficulty in clinical diagnosis of AD. Methodology is advancing quickly, however, and prospects of definitive answers within the next few years are real.

Even if a specific genetic cause is demonstrated, this will leave unanswered many questions regarding the cause and mechanisms of AD. Principal among these is the question of why the expression of a supposed AD genotype should be delayed for over seventy-five years after birth. An understanding of the causes of this delay could result in specific interventions that might result in a further delay of several years. Such a delay would have the remarkable consequence of greatly reducing the prevalence of AD, as many more predisposed individuals would die of other illnesses while their predisposition to AD remained unexpressed.

Even now the actual impact of any presumed genetic cause of AD is severely lessened by death from other causes. By comparing the curve of figure 3.2 with known current population survival characteristics, it may be estimated that only about one-third of those with a presumptive predisposition to AD will develop it within their natural lifetime. If AD were attributable to an autosomal-dominant gene, the actual risk of developing it would then be on the order of 17 percent (one in six) for first-degree relatives of carefully diagnosed AD probands. (It will be considerably lower when more commonly applied clinical diagnostic criteria are used.) While hardly reassuring, this risk is far lower than that in well-known autosomal-dominant genetic disorders such as Huntington's disease. Thus, further analyses of the clinical genetics of AD may offer the prospect of a beneficial increase in understanding (and possibly treatment) of its underlying mechanisms, while lacking the dire prognostic consequences usually associated with genetic illnesses.

Glossary

epidemiology the study of the distribution and determinants of diseases and injuries in human populations.

first-degree relative parent, sibling, or offspring (a blood relation).

genetics the branch of science that deals with heredity (the transmission of characteristics from parent to offspring).

genotype the genetic constitution of an individual.

incidence the rate of appearance of new cases of a disease in a population over a period of time.

pedigree a register recording a line of ancestors (a family tree).

phenotype a category or group to which an individual may be assigned on the basis of one or more observable characteristics that may reflect genetic variation.

prevalence the proportion of people in a population who have the disease at a given time.

proband or index cases identified individuals diagnosed with the disease.

risk factors factors whose presence is associated with an increased probability that disease will develop later on.

References

General

Breitner, J. C. S. 1987. Genetic factors in the etiology of Alzheimer's disease. In *American College of Neuropsychopharmacology: a third generation of progress,* ed. H. Y. Meltzer. New York: Raven Press.

Heston, L. L., and White, J. A. 1983. *Dementia: A practical guide to Alzheimer's Disease and related illness.* New York: W. H. Freeman & Co.

McKhann, G. et al. 1984. Clinical diagnosis of Alzheimer's disease: Report of the NINCDS-ADRDA Work Group under the auspices of Department of Health and Human Services Task Force on Alzheimer's Disease. *Neurology* 34:939–44.

Tomlinson, B. E. 1982. Plaques, tangles and Alzheimer's disease. *Psychol. Med.* 12:449–59.

Specific Studies

Breitner, J. C. S., and Folstein, M. F. 1984. Familial Alzheimer dementia: a prevalent disorder with specific clinical features. *Psychol. Med.* 14:63–80.

Heston, L. L. et al. 1981. Dementia of the Alzheimer type: Clinical genetics, natural history and associated conditions. *Arch. Gen. Psychiatry* 38:1085–90.

Heyman, A. et al. 1983. Alzheimer's disease: genetic aspects and associated clinical disorders. *Ann. Neurol.* 14:507–15.

Kallmann, F. J., and Sander, G. 1949. Twin studies on senescence. *Am J. Psychiatry* 106:29–36.

Mohs, R. C., Breitner, J. C. S., Silverman, J. M., and Davis, K. L. 1987. Alzheimer's disease: Morbid risk among first-degree relatives approximates 50% by ninety years of age. *Arch. Gen. Psychiatry*, 44: 405–8.

Nee, L. E., et al. 1983. A Family with Histologically Confirmed Alzheimer's Disease. *Arch. Neurol.* 40:203–8.

CHAPTER FOUR

Treatment Strategies: Present and Future

Leon J. Thal, M.D.

Rationale for Treatment

ALZHEIMER'S DISEASE (AD) IS a disorder with an increasing rate of occurrence among the elderly. Thus, as the population ages, the number of individuals afflicted with this disorder will continue to increase. In the 1970s it was first realized that memory impairment is not an inevitable consequence of the aging process. A second important discovery was that younger individuals with AD (formerly called presenile dementia) and older individuals with senile dementia have the same pathological changes in their brains. This suggests that presenile and senile dementia represent a single disease. Today there are more than two million people in the United States who have AD or senile dementia of the Alzheimer type. Recent advances in our understanding of the disease, and the knowledge that this disorder is a major public health issue, have led to a marked increase in research in an attempt to find both the cause and treatment of this disorder.

During the last twenty-five years, many different medications have been tested as potential treatments for this disorder. Early treatment trials were largely empirical; that is, drugs were developed in the laboratory based on their ability to improve memory in animals whose memory had been disrupted by drugs or electroconvulsive treatment. Following safety studies in animals, these compounds were then tested for efficacy in humans. Alternatively, some compounds were found to enhance cognition (overall knowledge) or memory when being tested for some other purpose.

For many years memory loss was considered to be a consequence of cerebral atherosclerosis or "hardening of the arteries of the brain." It is now known that this is not the case. While blood flow to the brain does decrease in AD, this decrease occurs as brain cells cease to function and die. The decrease in blood flow that results is a secondary event rather than the cause of the dementia. Additionally, the brain is extremely efficient at removing oxygen from blood. Therefore, even with the modest decrease in blood flow, brain tissue in AD does not lack oxygen. Nevertheless, many of these facts were not known until fairly recently, and many early pharmacological treatments for AD centered around the use of vasodilators, compounds designed to increase blood flow by dilating blood vessels.

In 1972 a new class of drugs known as nootropic agents was described by scientists. Nootropics are believed to improve mental functioning, presumably by enhancing metabolic processes within the brain. These compounds produce such effects in experimental animals without producing the side effects common with psychoactive drugs, such as sedation, sleep, or stiffness. These compounds are quite safe and continue to undergo considerable clinical testing.

In 1976 three independent groups of investigators made a very important neurochemical discovery in the brains of deceased Alzheimer patients. These research groups demonstrated a marked loss of choline acetyltransferase, the enzyme

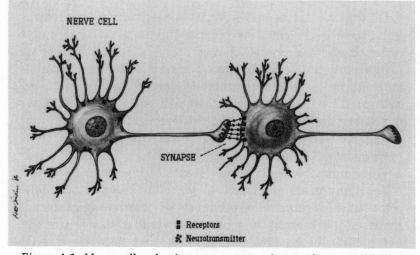

NERVE CELL

SYNAPSE

∎ Receptors
✻ Neurotransmitter

Figure 4.1. Nerve cells releasing a neurotransmitter such as acetylcholine that migrates across the space called a synapse and attaches to a specialized region on the next cell, called a receptor.

that makes acetylcholine (a chemical messenger used to transmit information between nerve cells) in the cortex of Alzheimer patients. This finding strongly suggested that there was a deficiency of acetylcholine in the subjects' brains. More important, the acetylcholine deficit was not present in all parts of the brain but appeared to occur most prominently in the cortex, the region of the brain responsible for such higher brain functions as memory, speech, and reasoning. This important finding was confirmed by many other investigators, and subsequent studies have shown that the loss of this enzyme is strongly correlated with the severity of memory loss in AD. This suggests that replacing the missing acetylcholine might improve memory.

Neurotransmitters normally function by being released from a nerve cell, migrating across a small space called a synapse and attaching to the next cell at a specialized region called a receptor (fig. 4.1). Different receptors recognize different neurotransmitters. In AD, the brain receptor for acetylcholine appears to be present in relatively normal numbers, which further suggests that if a replacement compound (called an agonist) for acetylcholine could be developed, its activity would imitate the action of acetylcholine, resulting in memory and cognitive improvement. With this knowledge, scientists have begun designing specific drugs to improve neurotransmission in this disorder. These compounds are designed to either increase the availability of acetylcholine or to mimic its actions in the brain.

In addition to changes in the cholinergic system, we now know that other neurotransmitter systems are also abnormal in AD. Smaller decreases in the neurotransmitters noradrenaline and serotonin have also been reported. Neuropeptides, an entirely new class of neurotransmitters, may also be involved in AD. The most important neuropeptide change has been the approximately 50 percent decrease in somatostatin in the cortex of Alzheimer patients.

It should be pointed out that neurotransmitter loss appears to be a consequence rather than a cause of the disease. That is, as various cells die, they lose their ability to produce normal quantities of neurotransmitter compounds. However, it is not believed that the loss of neurotransmitter material is responsible for cell death. Still, the pattern of neurotransmitter loss provides important clues about the disease. For example, while the neuropeptide somatostatin is diminished in Alzheimer patients, many other peptides that also act as neurotransmitter substances are present in normal concentrations in these patients, which suggests that not all classes of cells undergo degeneration in this disorder.

Review of Noncholinergic Drugs

Currently, only a small number of drugs are clinically available for the treatment of intellectual dysfunction (table 4.1). These include three vasodilators: Cyclospasmol, Pavabid, and

Table 4.1

Drugs Currently Used in the United States to Treat Cognitive Dysfunction

VASODILATORS	METABOLIC ENHANCERS—VASODILATORS
Cyclospasmol	Hydergine
Pavabid	
Vasodilan	

Experimental Agents Undergoing Testing as Possible Cognitive Enhancers in Alzheimer's Disease

EXPERIMENTAL NOOTROPIC AGENTS	CHOLINERGIC AGENTS
Praxilene	Acetylcholine precursors
Piracetam	choline
Oxiracetam	lecithin
Pramiracetam	Cholinesterase inhibitors
CI 911	physostigmine
PEPTIDES	tetrahydroaminoacridine
ACTH 4-10	Agonists
ORG 2766 (ACTH analog 4–9)	arecoline
	RS 86
Vasopressin, DDAVP, DGAVP	bethanechol
	MISCELLANEOUS
Naloxone, naltrexone	Zimelidine
L 363586 (somatostatin analog)	Nimodipine
	Vinpocetine
	Chelating agents

Vasodilan. Although multiple studies have been carried out with these compounds, clinically significant improvement in demented patients has not been demonstrated.

Hydergine, an ergot alkaloid believed to be both a metabolic enhancer and a vasodilator, is now the most widely used medication for treating AD. It has been subjected to more than twenty controlled clinical trials. Virtually all of these trials have noted statistically significant improvement in such behavioral or psychological functions as sociability, memory, confusion, and mood. Most studies using Hydergine have used either the physician's overall impression or a behavioral rating scale to determine drug usefulness. Therefore, it is not certain whether Hydergine exerts its effect by improving memory or behavior. It is also not clear whether the changes produced by Hydergine are clinically meaningful in the majority of patients. Many clinicians have reported an occasional dramatic response to this compound, which suggests that at least a portion of the population might benefit from this drug. Side effects from Hydergine are uncommon, with rare occurrences of headache or facial flushing.

The vasodilators and the metabolic enhancer Hydergine are the only drugs licensed in the United States for the treatment of cognitive deficits. All other agents that are undergoing clinical testing are experimental. None have been proved to be effective and safe for the treatment of cognitive deficits. Some are marketed for other indications; the majority are entirely experimental compounds, with proof of efficacy yet to be determined.

A second major group of noncholinergic medications are the nootropic agents. They are believed to improve function without producing any of the side effects characteristic of traditional psychoactive medications. In animals, they have been reported to protect against electroshock-induced amnesia, while in humans they have been reported to enhance verbal learning dyslexia and to improve alertness and IQ scores in elderly individuals with schizophrenia and affective disorders. Small investigator-sponsored trials of these compounds in AD in the United States have resulted in conflicting reports of either increased memory, improved mood, or no change. Many of these compounds have undergone extensive clinical testing in the United States as part of multicenter double-blind placebo-controlled clinical trials. Trials of Pramiracetam and CI 911 have been completed. Despite preliminary data suggesting effectiveness based on open studies, none of these agents has been shown to be effective in Alzheimer patients in these carefully controlled double-blind studies.

Another nootropic agent, Piracetam, has undergone limited testing both alone and in combination with choline. Preliminary data indicate that the combination of these two drugs might produce a synergistic effect, that is, a greater response than one would see by simply adding the effect of the two drugs together. However, a large-scale double-blind study comparing Piracetam and choline to a placebo has not yet been carried out.

Several peptides, or small proteins, have also been tested in treating AD. These include several fragments of a steroid hormone called adrenocorticotrophic hormone (ACTH), as well as vasopressin, and a series of related compounds (DDAVP, DGAVP). These agents appear to improve attention and mood rather than learning and memory, however, and the effects are small and difficult to reproduce. In general, neuropeptides must be administered by injection or intranasally. Side effects consist of salt and fluid retention.

A single recent study of considerable interest suggested that naloxone, a drug known to counteract the effect of opiates (an opiate antagonist), might be useful in the treatment of AD. However, several subsequent studies have failed to demonstrate a positive effect on memory. Still, based on both human and animal studies, it appears that naloxone and other opiate antagonists may improve attention and concentration. Studies are currently under way using naltrexone, an orally administered opiate antagonist, to determine if this form of therapy is useful in Alzheimer patients. To date, preliminary results have been negative with respect to memory enhancement.

Because the neuropeptide somatostatin shows the greatest decrease in the brains of Alzheimer patients, a trial of somatostatin would be of major clinical interest. However, somatostatin is a peptide that cannot be administered orally and will not cross the blood-brain barrier even when administered intravenously. One study used a somatostatin analog, L 363586, but the results of careful clinical testing demonstrated no effect in patients with mild AD. However, the drug was not present in cerebrospinal fluid, which suggests that this compound failed to cross the blood-brain barrier and therefore probably never reached the brain. It is too early to tell whether treatment with a somatostatinlike compound that enters the brain might result in cognitive improvement in Alzheimer patients.

Several other interesting drugs have been investigated within the past several years. One study examined the effects of a compound called zimelidine, which is known to increase serotonin availability to the brain. This drug was tried in Alzheimer patients, whose brains are known to have reduced serotonin levels. The trial results, however, were negative. Nimodipine, a calcium channel blocker, has recently been tested, based on the belief that preventing the entry of calcium into nerve cells might slow the death of cells during the disease process. The initial phase of testing has been completed, and the preliminary data appear negative. Vinpocetine, a drug known to increase glucose use in the brain, as well as blood flow, is currently undergoing a multicenter trial in the United States for individuals with dementia secondary to multiple strokes. Preliminary results have not been published but appear to be promising. The drug is currently also undergoing testing in patients with AD.

Aluminum salts have been found in elevated concentrations in the brains of Alzheimer patients by some, but not all, investigators. However, it is not known if aluminum causes cell death or whether aluminum simply deposits in cells that are dying because the cell is unable to keep the aluminum out. Despite this uncertainty regarding the role of aluminum, some individuals have been treated with chelating agents in an attempt to remove metals, such as aluminum, from brain cells. There are no published controlled reports substantiating efficacy for this form of therapy.

Cholinergic Strategies

A large amount of data has accumulated over the years implicating the cholinergic division of the nervous system in memory disorders. In the 1930s a drug called scopolamine was commonly used in conjunction with a pain medication to deaden pain during labor and delivery. Women treated with this combination of drugs not only had pain relief but often failed to remember the events of delivery. Scopolamine is known to prevent the normal action of the neurotransmitter acetylcholine. In the early 1970s it was administered to young healthy college students and induced memory disruption, which was then reversed by administering the drug physostigmine, a compound that increases the availability of acetylcholine. Many animal experiments carried out in the 1970s also confirmed that damage to certain neurons containing acetylcholine resulted in impairment of memory and spatial relations. Finally, in the middle to late 1970s, the loss of acetylcholine-containing neurons was demonstrated in the brains of Alzheimer patients. These observations strongly suggested that the loss of acetylcholine in Alzheimer patients led to memory loss. Clinicians began to develop strategies to replace this missing neurotransmitter.

Early drug trials attempted to increase brain acetylcholine content by the administration of either oral choline or lecithin. This form of treatment is known as precursor replacement therapy. It is based on the assumption that by administering a neurotransmitter precursor, a chemical reaction will result, converting swallowed choline into acetylcholine. To date, more than twenty-five studies have been carried out using either choline chloride in doses of up to 16 grams per day or lecithin in doses ranging up to 100 grams per day. While initial open studies suggested mild improvement in some patients, all of the double-blind studies have failed to demonstrate improvement.

Why has this form of therapy failed? There are several possible explanations. First, subsequent work in animals has failed to demonstrate that the administration of choline or lecithin can significantly increase brain acetylcholine levels. Second, since in AD there is an inadequate amount of the enzyme necessary to convert choline into acetylcholine, the diseased brain may not be capable of producing more acetylcholine.

The second strategy employed was the use of an inhibitor designed to prevent the breakdown of the neurotransmitter acetylcholine by the enzyme cholinesterase. With these compounds, levels of acetylcholine in the brain rise because destruction of the neurotransmitter has been slowed. Several early studies were carried out with injectable physostigmine, demonstrating small improvements in memory and spatial relations. Seven double-blind studies have now been carried out using oral physostigmine. Four of these studies have shown that physostigmine can produce beneficial effects on memory and on some behavioral tasks. However, the degree of improvement demonstrated in each of these studies has been only very modest. While many patients improve on testing performed in the laboratory, the improvements are often quite small and not of sufficient magnitude to result in functional improvement in the home environment. Approximately one-third of treated patients in the positive studies have small degrees of improvement that were clearly apparent to family members. However, in no instance was an individual restored to normal health.

The response to oral physostigmine is not uniform. Patients with mild to moderate dementia appear to respond better than those with severe dementia. The dose is also important. In the positive studies, higher doses were employed. The use of high-dose oral physostigmine, however, can result in many side effects, including nausea, vomiting, and change in blood pressure and pulse rate. In addition, after a single dose the medication remains in the body for less than two hours, making multiple repeated doses necessary. In its present form it has no major clinical use, but the development of a timed-release formulation might greatly enhance its clinical utility.

A second, longer-acting cholinesterase inhibitor called tetrahydroaminoacridine (THA) has also undergone limited testing in clinical trials. One early trial was positive, while the other was negative. In 1986 a third small clinical trial was published that reported functional improvement in sixteen of seventeen Alzheimer patients treated with higher doses of THA. Additional clinical trials of THA will begin in early 1987.

Cholinergic agonists, compounds that mimic the action of acetylcholine, have structures similar to that of acetylcholine. The receptor of acetylcholine is tricked into believing that the agonist is acetylcholine. Because this receptor appears to be intact in AD, direct stimulation of the receptor seems like a very promising approach for therapeutic intervention. Acetylcholine itself is not a useful compound, because it is destroyed when given orally and remains active in the body for only minutes after intravenous administration. What is needed is a cholinergic agonist that can be given orally, remain in the body for several hours, and stimulate only brain acetylcholine receptors but not acetylcholine receptors in the rest of the body. Such a compound would be useful in reducing side effects such as sweating, nausea, or vomiting. Unfortunately, only a very few cholinergic agonists exist that are capable of entering the brain, one of which is arecoline. This compound has been tried, and some improvement has been demonstrated in Alzheimer patients using small intravenous doses. However, major side effects (including sweating and vomiting) and the need for intravenous administration limit its usefulness. A second orally active cholinergic agonist, RS 86, is currently being tested in a small number of patients. A limited degree of improvement in memory and word fluency was noted in some patients. Once again, many of them experienced side effects, including sweating, chills, and flushing. Several clinical trials with this compound are still under way, and its efficacy remains unknown, but it is clear that the ideal cholinergic agonist remains to be discovered.

A summary of the drugs and agents discussed appears in table 4.1.

Delivery Systems

The delivery of drugs to the central nervous system is a formidable problem. Some compounds cannot be given orally because they are destroyed by acid in the digestive tract, others are poorly absorbed, some are active for only brief periods and require frequent administration, while others fail to cross the blood-brain barrier and do not reach the intended site of action. A number of strategies have been developed to deal with each of these problems. In some instances it is possible to change the chemical nature of the molecule to make it resistant to breakdown by stomach acids without destroying the activity of the drug. Other alternate routes for administering drugs have been developed, including the use of a buccal preparation, that is, the placement of a tablet on a person's gums, to allow for slow, continuous release. This approach has recently been used to develop a form of morphine for relief of chronic pain instead of resorting to frequent injections. A second approach has been administering drugs by absorption through the skin (called transdermal). Preparations of nitroglycerin for the treatment of angina and of scopolamine for the treatment of motion sickness are now available in transdermal preparations that bypass the stomach and allow for very slow, continuous release. Several drugs are currently being prepared as controlled-release formulations to sustain blood levels on only two or three tablets per day.

There are several medications used to treat certain forms of cancer that need to be delivered to the brain but are blocked when given intravenously because of the blood-brain barrier. These medications are sometimes delivered directly to the brain by using a small pump implanted under the skin and connected to a small catheter located in a brain cavity that contains cerebrospinal fluid. Using this system, the drug is released directly into the cerebrospinal fluid and absorbed by the brain, thereby bypassing the blood-brain barrier. When empty, the pump can be refilled by injecting additional drug into a reservoir located under the skin. Several years ago, four Alzheimer patients received a cholinergic agonist, called bethanechol, by use of this implantable pump. The preliminary report from this study was mildly encouraging, and a multicenter trial has been undertaken to evaluate this form of therapy. Approximately eighty patients are now enrolled in studies of bethanechol in the United States. Results of this clinical trial have not been published, but reports presented at a number of meetings indicate uncertainty regarding patient improvement with this form of therapy. Additionally, implanting the pump is a major surgical procedure, and there have been a number of serious complications, including infection, seizures, hemorrhage, and death. The final results of this important clinical trial are eagerly awaited.

Brain-Cell Implants

The idea of a brain-cell implant may seem like science fiction, but in 1982 two patients with severe Parkinson's disease, a disorder characterized by a loss of the neurotransmitter dopamine, underwent brain implantation, when they were no longer responding to conventional treatment. Tissue known to produce dopamine was removed from the adrenal gland of each patient and grafted deep within their respective brains. Both patients showed transient improvement in symptoms for a matter of days. Although their clinical improvement was not maintained, this procedure demonstrated the technical feasibility of using brain implants to treat neurological illness. Recently, Parkinsonian patients in Mexico were reported to improve significantly after adrenal transplant surgery. In AD there is a marked degeneration of acetylcholine-containing cells. It may be feasible to improve the functioning of the cholinergic system by inserting grafts containing acetylcholine-producing neurons.

Additional Future Treatment Strategies

In addition to the use of brain grafts, it may be possible to halt the degeneration of nerve cells in Alzheimer individuals. A peptide called nerve growth factor (NGF) has recently been shown to increase concentrations of the enzyme that produces acetylcholine when injected into the brains of newborn rats. Some acetylcholine-containing neurons in the brain appear to require a continuing source of NGF to survive. If acetylcholine-containing nerve cells do not have a continuing source of NGF, they degenerate and die. Several investigators have now demonstrated that administering NGF into the brains of rats can prevent the death of acetylcholine-containing neurons after they have been physically damaged. Rats with certain types of brain lesions demonstrate deficits in memory and learning and serve as a model for AD. Current investigations are under way to determine if the administration of NGF can counteract these learning deficits by preventing loss of the neurons. Additionally, grafting work in animals has demonstrated that after removal of the hippocampus, a region of the brain required for normal memory, the placement of a cholinergic graft can restore memory and spatial relations. These observations suggest that either NGF or cholinergic implants, or a combination of both, may be useful in treating Alzheimer patients in the future. While the use of graft techniques for the treatment of AD is far off, the administration of NGF by an implantable pump is a form of treatment that might reach clinical testing within the next several years.

Treatment of Associated Symptoms

The treatment of associated symptoms such as anxiety, agitation, sleep disturbance, and depression remains extremely important in the overall management of the Alzheimer patient and is discussed in chapter 9. Treatment of these symptoms should be undertaken in all patients whose behavior problems interfere with their own well-being or that of their family caregivers. Medications for these conditions are accepted treatments.

In summary, during the previous ten years tremendous strides have been made in diagnosing and understanding AD. In the early 1970s there were very few investigators involved in research or treatment of AD. However, modern biochemical techniques have taught us a great deal about the neurochemical alterations of the disorder. As a consequence, a whole host of new therapeutic approaches have been explored. During the next decade the advances made in cellular neurobiology will also be applied to the study of this disease. Although we do not yet have an adequate treatment or cure, there are many hopeful avenues currently being explored. Clearly, research along two lines is required. First, researchers are addressing the immediate need to develop a treatment for those already afflicted with the disorder. It is clear that in modern medicine we are often able to treat diseases without fully understanding their cause. Thus, we can treat Parkinson's disease with L-dopa and diabetes with insulin without knowing the cause of either disease. The second line of research continues the search for the cause of AD, for only then will we develop an effective therapy and ultimately a means of prevention.

Glossary

acetylcholine a chemical messenger used by many brain cells to transmit information.

agonist a compound that has the same action as the parent compound.

antagonist a compound that blocks the action of the parent compound.

blood-brain barrier a specialized system within blood vessels of the brain designed to keep undesirable chemicals out of the brain.

choline acetyltransferase a compound known as an enzyme, the presence of which is required to make acetylcholine from choline.

cognition knowledge in the broadest sense.

cortex the outer layer of the brain.

double-blind placebo-controlled study a study in which neither the patient nor the investigator is aware of which patients are on placebo and which are on active drug.

neuropeptides compounds made up of proteins that serve as neurotransmitters in the brain.

neurotransmitters chemicals released by the brain to communicate with other nerve cells. Acetylcholine and dopamine are two neurotransmitters.

nootropic drugs compounds producing cognitive effects in animals that do not produce undesirable side effects.

placebo an inactive compound, usually sugar or starch.

psychoactive active on the mind.

receptor that portion of the cell membrane, or outer lining, that is specialized to recognize and respond to individual neurotransmitters.

somatostatin a neuropeptide that is decreased in the brains of Alzheimer patients.

vasodilators compounds that increase blood flow by increasing the diameter of blood vessels.

References

Alzheimer's disease: a report of progress in research. 1982. In *Aging*, vol. 19, ed. S. Corkin et al. New York: Raven Press.

Bartus, R. et al. 1982. The cholinergic hypotheses of geriatric memory dysfunction. *Science* 217:408–17.

Crook, T., and Gershon, S., eds. 1981. *Strategies for the development of an effective treatment for senile dementia.* New Canaan, Conn.: Mark Powley Associates, Inc.

Katzman, R. 1986. Alzheimer's disease. *N. Engl. J. Med.* 314:964–73. (Available through ADRDA)

Wurtman, R. J. 1985. Alzheimer's disease. *Scientific American* 252:62–66, 71–74. (Available through ADRDA)

PART II

How to Cope

CHAPTER FIVE

A Crisis as a Challenge

Marcella Bakur Weiner, Ed.D.

THE SAYING "WHEN LIFE HANDS you lemons, make lemonade" sounds simplistic. Yet, as with many simple facts of life, truths exist. While we cannot manipulate life to our benefit as much as we would like, we can make a difficult or intolerable situation better. Sometimes that kind of position allows us to recognize a part of ourselves that was, until the time of crisis, unknown to us. It is as though a hidden, unrevealed piece of who we are suddenly pushes forward, raises its hand, and shouts, "Here I am." People who have that positive piece inside themselves (and most of us do!) rise to the critical situation, overcome it, and create a new way of living, obliterating much of the pain and misery of everyday life with someone with Alzheimer's disease (AD).

Laura D. did just that. An active, vibrant woman who had been a librarian for many years, she was now, at seventy-eight, in her third marriage. It was her best one; her two former marriages had ended in divorce after years of turmoil. Her third marriage had lasted the longest, and she was, simply, happy. Ed was a wonderful man, she felt. Sensitive to her needs and happy to have found a second wife he loved after he'd been widowed, he was attentive to her, a good companion and friend, and accepting and glad for the fact that he now also had a grown stepson, since he had been childless. Retired, Laura and Ed could now spend as much time as they liked together, and that is exactly what they did. Financially comfortable, if not wealthy, they did some traveling, were active in some community groups, did some visiting, and spent much time alone, glad to be with each other.

Then came the lemons—a barrelful. Ed started to change, showing all the usual signs associated with the onset of AD. Typical of all family members in that situation, Laura was greatly distressed, fighting the tremendous sense of loss—the loss of Ed as he had been—and her own despair, another sense of loss within herself as she had known *herself* to be! After the diagnosis had been confirmed, she tried, for a long time, to cope with the situation by keeping Ed at home. The usual, "No nursing home for my darling," was often heard, and I, her therapist, to whom she had come for relief and as a way of strengthening herself, was in agreement with her feelings. Since Laura wished to keep Ed at home and could manage, it seemed plausible. And then it no longer was possible. Ed's downhill path was progressing rapidly, and Laura and her hired help could no longer keep up with his accelerated deterioration. How many times, she asked me, would she be able to continue to clean up all the feces in the bed, on the carpets, on the chairs? I gently suggested she think about placement, since she was evidently feeling hopeless and I was concerned for her. As with many caring people, Laura responded to the suggestion with two feelings—guilt and relief—for, indeed, she felt she could no longer cope. She acted on the suggestion as a way of both saving herself and doing the best for Ed.

She stayed in therapy to get the soothing, comfort, and

caring she seemed to need. She thrived and, most important, survived. Yet the nagging sense of "I've put him away"
stayed with her. Session after therapy session dealt with her
life with Ed: how happy she was to have found him, the
early years, the middle years—and then the beginning of
the end. She spoke eloquently, with feeling and awareness.
I suggested she jot down some of her ideas. She began to
do so, at first bringing in a dream or fragment of a dream,
then a waking dream, then some pieces of memory from
last year, twenty years ago, forty years ago, all part of the
"album of her mind," as we both began to call it. It was a
rich album, full of color and texture, showing many years of
living, thinking, and feeling. It also did something most important for Laura: it gave her a chance to do her own life
review and come to terms with herself. As with most normal, healthy, and functioning persons, the ability to stand
off a bit, away from ourselves, looking at ourselves from a
small distance (but with empathy!), gives us a new perspective. It is like looking at the whole road one is traveling on,
noticing every rock, flower springing out from an unlikely
place, frog camouflaged in his green, and the ways in which
the road goes straight or suddenly curves. It is a way of
reflecting on and integrating one's experiences in living. Laura
was doing just that. Her writing was simple but profound.
After a short while, each piece of her life's history became a
small story, with a real beginning, middle, and end. I suggested to her that perhaps she would like to write short stories or even a book. "Do you think I could?" she asked one
day with surprise and joy. "Why not?" I responded. "That's
what you've been doing, anyway, isn't it?" She agreed.

Ed was a most definite part of all her stories. Now not
only in her mind, he had been transcribed onto paper, for
her, for me, perhaps for others, to see and learn about. Most
urgently, she felt she wanted to share both the happiness
and the pain she had experienced with him. If others could
read of her feelings, her actions, perhaps they, too, could

be helped. Certainly putting all of it on paper was helping her. Her despair now had a cover, like a warm comforter on a hard bed, for radiance was visible. While the frequent visits to Ed at his nursing home left her depleted, her solace was her own self, her own writing, her own self-soothing. Each visit was followed by some new insight, some new awareness of her situation—or a long-ago memory now unplugged and put on paper. She was blossoming.

Now eighty-one, she is still blooming, still writing. She has just completed her book, an autobiography, an ordering of her life of eighty-one years. She is in therapy but not on a continuous basis. She comes, as she says, "when I need a booster shot," but that, too, has become more and more infrequent. Her literary agent (for now she has one) thinks her book will make an important contribution. Laura and I certainly hope so. But even if not, Laura, by writing that book, has contributed—to herself. The lemons have indeed produced barrels of the richest lemonade. For sale or not, it's great for drinking!

One of her poems appears below. It is a moving experience of living with an AD victim whom one loves. In order to protect her, we have not used her real name. But, hopefully, you will recognize it as "Laura D.'s" when it does appear, someday, in her very own book.

To You

I called and no one answered;
I cried and no one heard,
As though you weren't listening,
For you gave me not a word.

We used to reach each other
In sentiment and deed,
And now when I address you,
You pay my heart no heed.

We used to burst with laughter
  At each other's gauche deport;
At jokes we giggled, smiled, or grinned;
  We enjoyed such fine rapport.

I try again, I whisper,
  I struggle to get close to you;
You look but hardly see me,
  Yet you know me, yes you do.

I take your hand, you clasp not mine
  The way you used to do;
No stirring warmth electrifies
  The touch of me to you.

I plant a kiss upon your lips
  So unresponsive now;
I tell you that I love you,
  You don't affirm that vow.

I throw my arms about you,
  You are flesh but not the man;
Yet I know you'd surely want me
  If your affliction we could ban.

It's despairing how you've changed, dear,
  Yet you need me as yesteryear;
I pray to God to help you
  While you've life and I'm still here.

CHAPTER SIX

Patients and Families: Impact and Long-Term-Management Implications

Miriam K. Aronson, Ed.D.

DEMENTING ILLNESS—A progressive decline in intellectual function and a decreasing ability to perform daily job and social activities—is a serious public health problem that currently affects four million Americans. Alzheimer's disease (AD) is the most common form of dementing illness, accounting for more than half of the cases of dementia, and is the embodiment of everyone's worst fears. Nobody wants to "lose their mind" or lose control over their thoughts, their actions, or their environment.

At this writing, there are probably more than four million older adults with some degree of difficulty in intellectual functions, such as memory, learning, and problem solving. Of these four million, one-third are so impaired that they can no longer manage without assistance in the simplest daily routine activities, such as eating, dressing, grooming, and toileting. If one thinks about the impact of this illness and estimates that each victim may have three close family members, the number of persons involved escalates rapidly to fifteen million.

In terms of human suffering, there is probably no greater affliction than for a person to deteriorate slowly and steadily over a period of years—perhaps five to ten or more—and for family and friends to watch a loved one do so. Mrs. Bobbie Glaze, a founder of the national Alzheimer's Disease and Related Disorders Association (ADRDA), described the ordeal of her husband's illness as "the funeral that never ends." Others have described the experience as living with a stranger, that is, a person different from their spouse or parent. Still others have described themselves as being in a state of limbo; they're neither wives nor widows, neither husbands nor widowers.

Most dementia victims reside in the community with their families. For every demented person in a nursing home, there are at least two persons with a similar degree of incapacity being maintained at home. Social and financial factors such as who is available to care for the patient, how much time and energy family caregivers can expend, and how much money is available for purchasing outside services when needed are more likely to determine whether and/or when someone is to be placed in an institution than the patient's actual degree of intellectual, social, or physical impairment.

The major care providers of dementia patients are family members. Families, in fact, provide 70 percent of all care received. Generally, married patients are cared for by their spouse, often with assistance from children—usually daughters and sometimes daughters-in-law. When patients are widowed, children may assume the caregiving responsibility. Since most AD patients are elderly, middle-aged children often must become the caregivers for their parents. These middle-aged children have been called "the sandwich generation" because they are caught between the competing demands of their own lives—that is, responsibility to their spouse, children, work demands—and the burdens of caring for a demented elderly parent.

The Stresses of Caregiving

The following excerpt from a letter highlights the plight of the family:

> I'm writing to you on behalf of my parents. They, themselves, are not afflicted with Alzheimer's disease, but they have been affected by it and I'd like to see them get some help before they are completely devastated by it.
>
> Five or six years ago my mom and dad were vibrant and their lives were joyful and fulfilling. They were the envy of all who knew them. My dad was sixty-five and my mom was a year or two younger. They enjoyed life to its fullest and never missed a single dance or neighborhood party.
>
> Then grandma came to live with them. Until then, grandma had been living in Florida with my mother's sister. Because of gross neglect, indifference, and a lot of ignorance, grandma's health had severely deteriorated and whatever savings she may have had were totally depleted. A family "conclave" was held and grandma was flown to New York to be with my mom and dad in what everyone thought would be her "dying days."
>
> With my mom's loving care, grandma made a remarkable—if not downright miraculous—comeback . . . physically, that is. . . . But as quickly as her physical well-being was restored, her mental faculties began to deteriorate.
>
> A year or two ago grandma suffered several "mini-strokes" that left her in almost as bad a physical condition as when she first arrived. Last Christmas I was able to see my folks for the first time in three to four years, and the toll that their dedicated service has taken alarmed me exceedingly.
>
> I fear for my parents' well-being. I know that grandma's days are numbered, and I admire my mom's devotion to her own mother. I understand my parents' aversion to having her committed to a nursing home, but I'm afraid it'll destroy THEM before it destroys HER.

Research has documented that the stresses of caregiving make caregivers themselves vulnerable to mental and physical problems. In a study of 100 caregiving spouses of AD patients done by Dr. Miriam Aronson at the Albert Einstein College of Medicine, we found an increase in the number of new cases of hypertension, increased occurrence of depression and of heart attack, when compared with general population figures for persons of similar age. Preliminary studies indicate that caregiver stress may be alleviated somewhat by use of services such as respite care (services that provide time away from caregiving) and family support groups; however, these services are not readily available in all areas and may be beyond the means of many families.

The symptoms of AD reflect the failing brain and cause marked changes in behavior and abilities. These changes impact on the patient's life-style, but even more important, they cause an ever-increasing need for supervision and care, usually by family members, who are the secondary victims of this disease. Table 6.1 contains a listing of symptoms and their impact on families.

Juliet Warshauer, a former president of the Westchester chapter of ADRDA, has described dealing with AD as being on an "emotional roller coaster." AD has some unique features that account for many of the emotional burdens that it imposes. What are they?

Emotional Costs

The patient looks "normal" and feels physically well. Certainly, at the beginning, it appears as though "just memory" is involved. Countless family members say, "He's healthy as can be except for his memory." The patient may be physically active and capable of chopping wood or jogging five miles but cannot perform a simple task such as preparing a cup of coffee, setting a table, or taking a telephone message. He or she seems to be quite sociable, to speak fairly well, and to remember old information but cannot remember what he or she ate five minutes ago. Does the patient have a se-

Table 6.1

Some Symptoms of Alzheimer's Disease and Their Manifestations in Routine Activities and Impact on Families

Symptom	Activity Impairment	Family Impact
1. Memory loss	Difficulty remembering names, events	May feel angry or abandoned when patient forgets them or does not acknowledge birthdays or holidays
	Difficulty remembering simple but important information such as removing a teapot from flame	May feel a need to restrict activities, supervise patient, or move patient to more structured environment, as they may have realistic fears for patient's safety
	Asking the same question over and over	May feel annoyed and harassed
2. Disorientation to time and place	Difficulty keeping appointments	May have to provide cues
	Difficulty finding one's way in familiar surroundings	May lose the only "driver"; may have to provide supervision

3. Disorientation to person	Misidentification of loved ones—calling spouse, children, by wrong names	May feel devastated and unappreciated
4. Visual-spatial problems	Difficulty operating even simple equipment, e.g., finding the knob on the radio or TV	Can't rely on patient for even simple tasks
	Difficulty finding one's way around a new environment, e.g., finding one's room in a hotel	Must think about changes in environment and sometimes change life-style
5. Language deficits	Difficulty saying what one wishes to say	May feel a wider communications gap as disease progresses
	Failing to initiate	May feel their world shrinking
	Difficulty following instructions	Patient increasingly dependent; caregiver frustrated

Table 6.1 (*cont.*)

Symptom	Activity Impairment	Family Impact
6. Calculation	Difficulty handling money	Person/family vulnerable to dishonesty
	Difficulty handling finances, e.g., balancing checkbook	May experience financial difficulties as a result of mishandling; potential embarrassment
7. Poor judgment	Inappropriate behavior	Embarrassment
	Sloppiness, carelessness	May be danger to self or others
8. Confusion	May misplace objects and then accuse others of stealing	May become angry at accusations
9. Personality change	May act differently from person he/she once was	May report "living with strangers"
10. Unpredictability	Erratic, impulsive, inappropriate behavior	May experience embarrassment

lective memory, remembering only what he or she wants to remember? How could this person be sick and look so well? It is a constant struggle for family and friends to deal rationally with the discrepancy between how a patient looks and how he or she functions.

The illness is insidious. Its onset is gradual and hard to pinpoint. Although there are generally no episodes of acute illness, the patient's symptoms become increasingly pronounced with time. It is difficult for families to deal with an illness that doesn't make you "sick" and that doesn't have symptoms you can recognize at the time. Furthermore, despite extensive efforts in public education, the illness still carries a stigma, perhaps because some of its behavioral manifestations mimic mental illness or perhaps because it has been associated with aging, which our society tends to treat negatively. It's hard to admit to a vague problem that, if identified, may cause other people to shun you.

Communication is another difficulty. Many patients experience word-finding problems, cannot seem to make the connections quickly enough to get his or her thoughts out in normal conversation, and may tend to withdraw socially to prevent embarrassment. Said one patient, "Every time I go to say something, someone's thought of it first. So I've become the silent partner, since I don't want to have egg on my face." This withdrawal may extend beyond stressful social situations as language skills become more impaired. Eventually the patient may lose his or her verbal skills, and ultimately the caregiver will lose all feedback from the patient. In most other illnesses, the patient is generally able to participate at least somewhat in his or her care and is able to acknowledge another's effort, saying, "Honey, I love you" or "Thank you for helping me." As AD progresses, the patient may become nonverbal and not be able to express anything at all. And, along the way, as a result of physical brain changes, the patient may develop paranoia, or suspiciousness, which may make things even worse. He or she may

demand: Why are you taking my money? Who is the intruder (often the very person who is totally devoted)? Why
is the food poisoned? What are you/they doing to me? It's
devastating for a caregiver to give unstintingly of himself or
herself and then to get criticism or outright hostility in return, but it happens.

AD involves a series of losses and protracted grieving. At
the time of diagnosis the patient may become depressed over
his or her losses of ability. This depression may continue
until later in the illness; however, as the illness progresses,
even the capacity to be depressed is lost. For the family
members it's much more painful. The grief goes on and on.
The decline of the patient is inexorable. Although with the
progression of the illness the person ultimately residing in
the body of the patient is entirely different from the original
person, the shell of a living person remains for a long time.
Therefore, there is no reference point for determining an end
to the mourning process until the patient's actual death,
which may be years subsequent to the victim's decline to a
nonfunctional being.

There are variations in how the patient functions from day
to day, sometimes from hour to hour or minute to minute.
The course of AD is generally downhill, and the patient will
be more noticeably impaired from one year to the next. On
rare occasions, a regressed, almost mute patient may make
an unexpectedly insightful remark, or a highly dependent
person may, atypically, dress or feed himself or herself. These
fluctuations may sometimes cause family members to deny
the severity of impairment and may even provide false hope.
They may cause families to doubt the wisdom of their decisions, for example, placing the patient in a nursing home.

Fluctuations may be more pronounced in multi-infarct dementia (MID), where "ministrokes" may be marked by the
patient's increased confusion or disorientation and may be
followed by periods of his or her improvement following the
downhill slide during the stroke. Multi-infarct patients also

tend to maintain more of their own personality for longer than AD patients and may retain some areas of strength but not others—for example, reading but not calculations.

Financial Costs

Aside from the emotional costs, the financial costs of AD may be staggering. The course of the illness may be five to ten years or more, of which five may require some kind of hands-on care, often skilled nursing care. If the average cost of skilled nursing care is $25,000 per year and the average patient requires five years of this type of care, the cost per patient just for nursing care can be as high as $125,000 per person, a tab that is well beyond the average pocketbook.

So what do families do? Some must eventually seek government subsidy in the form of Medicaid. It sounds simple, but actually this subsidy becomes readily available only when financial resources have become depleted, something that happens all too frequently to the families of Alzheimer patients. This is because Medicare, the system based on Social Security, which is widely available, generally does not cover nursing-home care for dementia victims. Similarly, although long-term-care insurance is becoming more available, dementia is often excluded, whether explicitly or through fine print.

Social Costs

The person with dementia is not the same as he or she once was, and there are associated changes in family and social relationships as well as life-style.

In those families in which there is a lot of denial regarding the illness, silence may develop and eventually estrangement, because needs cannot be discussed and problems solved collaboratively. Rather, anger and resentment may fill the gaps created by silence. The primary caregiver may resent the isolation. Other relatives may be angry at the primary caregiver for his or her inattention. Those who do not see the patient regularly may be fooled by preserved social skills that are exhibited on occasional visits with the patient, and may be wondering what all the fuss is about and why the caregiver is so upset. Further, dementia makes poor relationships worse and may strain good ones, so that old rivalries and points of contention may resurface.

Invariably, there will be role changes as the AD patient becomes less able to function independently. But we're talking about more than a role change when a person becomes a caregiver. Caregiving responsibilities are elastic, ever-expanding. As these new responsibilities increase, new roles accumulate and, in fact, eventually crowd out the other roles of the caregiving individual, who will eventually experience a loss of personal freedom and perhaps a loss of life opportunities.

As the patient's social skills deteriorate, he or she may no longer be able to be a good companion. Consequently, the well spouse may no longer fit well into the "couple's world" and may feel awkward with friends. As a result, the well spouse may become increasingly lonely.

Relationships with friends often change. Since both spouses are no longer able to participate in the same activities as before the illness, social engagements diminish. One AD caregiver recounts how her circle of friends shrank as her husband's illness progressed and how she found herself making "Alzheimer friends" through disease-related activities such as support groups and fund-raising. She finds her new friends interesting and stimulating—and a big comfort.

Changes in Life-style

AD may necessitate extensive changes in life-style. As time goes by, the patient may become increasingly dependent upon the well spouse, causing the well spouse to lead a more constricted life, focusing on the survival needs of the patient. The caregiver may have little or no leisure time or opportunity for recreation. Eventually, spouses may need to live apart.

Financial constraints may also change the quality of life, particularly if income is reduced because the caregiver is forced to leave his or her job or because the patient was the primary breadwinner. Likewise, if funds are spent on outside help, there may be less discretionary money for little luxuries and indulgences.

CESSATION OF DRIVING

With the increasing impairment in judgment that develops in AD, and the difficulties with visual and spatial coordination, the patient will need to stop driving a car. If the patient is the only driver in the household, the change may have a profound impact on everybody. Clearly, it would be advisable for the well spouse to get a driver's license. A wife of an AD victim who recognized that she would be immobile if she didn't learn how to drive got her driver's license at age sixty-five and appreciates the freedom and opportunity this new skill has afforded her. It is strongly urged that alternate means of transportation be provided for the person who must stop driving.

TRAVEL

Travel and vacation plans may have to be rethought. While changes in routine and time away may be necessary for the well spouse or other caregiving relatives, change may create confusion and disorientation for the patient. Thus, for those families who have two homes and are accustomed to traveling back and forth, it may become necessary to limit the trips. At first, families might spend two or three weeks or more at a time at the vacation home and eventually may decide on one primary residence for the patient, where he or she can have as many consistent environmental cues as possible.

Vacations may also have to be rethought. For the mildly affected patient, it may be wise to take vacations that were planned for the future, since as the disease progresses, the patient may become less able to appreciate or even comprehend certain experiences. The patient will usually do best with a vacation in a single place, involving familiar activities. For example, a patient who has always enjoyed the beach and swimming might appreciate a week or more at the shore.

Embarrassment

Early in the course of the disease, the patient is aware that something bad is happening to him or her. He or she may experience embarrassment at the inability to participate fully in social situations or to meet former standards of job performance. These patients often become depressed over their declining abilities. Mercifully for the patient, as this cruel, unrelenting dementia progresses, the patient's insight becomes diminished, and he or she may lose the capacity for embarrassment. Unfortunately, the potential for embarrassment is constantly there for the family.

Imagine yourself and your spouse at a dinner party at a friend's house in the company of friends, neighbors, and business acquaintances. Imagine your embarrassment when your spouse tastes the food and announces loudly, "I don't like it" or "I don't want it" or "Take this away." And imagine that he becomes more insistent and even agitated as you try to dissuade him quietly. You're so humiliated that you'd like to crawl under the table. Instead, you make a quick exit and go home early. You wonder how you will ever face these people again. . . .

Imagine that your husband, a successful accountant, has always taken care of the finances and has done it well. The checkbook was always balanced, the investments thrived, and the bills were paid on time. Suddenly you get a notice from the bank that several checks have bounced—a bank mistake, you're sure; but after you do some inquiring, you discover that it's really happening. Your finances are in disarray. You're shocked. After all, your credit rating has always been impeccable. Then you get a notice that your electricity will be shut off for nonpayment of several bills. Impossible, you hope, but again true. Now you're embarrassed—what do people think of us, of me? How can this be explained to others? How can I restore my credibility? How can I prevent this from happening again? How do I confront my husband about my having to assume his accustomed role?

Imagine that your wife calls the police upon your return from work and tells them "there is an intruder in the house." How ashamed you feel as you explain that you're her loving husband who takes good care of her day in and day out and now she misidentifies you when you come home.

If you have children at home, you must contend not only with your feelings but also with theirs. As we all have observed, teenagers are extremely sensitive to peer pressures and want to be like their friends. Unfortunately for children of a dementing parent, family life is not the same as it once was or as it is for friends and neighbors. Dad or Mom is, in fact, different and may behave peculiarly at times. These times are unpredictable, and odd behaviors may occur just when friends are in the house. Dad or Mom may insist on wearing three shirts that day or dirty old slippers or may carry a shopping bag filled with junk around the house. Or worse yet, Dad or Mom may actually get into fights with the children's friends over issues such as sitting in a particular chair, using the video games, or watching a particular TV program. The children may deal with their embarrassment by not inviting friends over at all, or they may spend less and less time at home themselves. They may or may not be able to express what's bothering them—more than likely they will "clam up" and avoid talking about their feelings.

Perspective

AD and related dementias have far-reaching implications for care. First and foremost is that caring for the patient means caring for both the patient and his or her family. We must never lose sight of this. Second, we are dealing with a long-term, progressive illness that requires varying kinds and amounts of services through its course. Third, since the family provides most of the care—and it is unlikely that this will change substantially—more extensive services must be made available to "support these supporters" in dealing with the burdens of caregiving. Fourth, a rational system for providing and financing long-term care must be developed. Fortunately, there is a national organization—ADRDA—working toward these goals. Clearly, until research provides us with the answers about cause and prevention, we will be faced with the task of stretching scarce resources among a growing patient group.

CHAPTER SEVEN

The Often Misunderstood Younger Alzheimer Victim: A Personal Perspective

Marion Roach

I WAS VERY ANGRY. I SAT THERE with the dictionary in my lap, wanting to hurl the book through the window. My mother put her hand on my shoulder. "What is it?" she asked, laughing the way only a mother can at her child's unbridled emotions. "Stupidity," I replied. "That's what it is, just stupidity. You're not getting senile, Ma. It's impossible."

In 1979 our family doctor suggested to me that my mother might be getting senile. I thought she was going mad. I called it madness—to myself. She kept losing her keys. She spoke in vague terms about wanting less responsibility for the day-to-day running of the house we shared. My father had died six months before, and I thought, at first, that she was just depressed. But then she disappeared for four days and had no idea where she'd gone. It terrified us both. She struggled with the names of familiar household objects like a semi-blind person reeling in the half-light of dusk. What began as a simple task of looking for her keys became a daily ritual of rage during which she would dump the contents of her purse on the floor and shriek that she was losing her mind.

My mother was fifty years old at the time. She was an only child, a good student, the recipient of a degree in journalism from the University of Colorado. She had been a newspaper reporter, a wife, a mother, a Girl Scout leader, and a visiting nurse/volunteer. After she raised my sister and me, she went back to school and got her master's degree in education. She became a teacher at a bilingual preschool on the Lower East Side of Manhattan, which is where she was working at the time the doctor suggested she was becoming "senile."

I was twenty-two at the time and working on a newspaper. We lived in the same house. We enjoyed one another's company. We were finally at that lovely, graceful period where we could go to museums and the ballet and play tennis and sail together and be equals, learning and sharing together, not one being taught, being watched over by the other. We were friends.

During the progression of her disease she became frightened, angry, paranoid, hostile, and incompetent. She became completely dependent on the aid of others. She could not be left alone. She became repetitive, confused, and agitated. She stopped reading. She couldn't form complete sentences. She spoke rapid gibberish. She lost all memory. She had to be fed, bathed, and dressed. She now lives in a nursing home where this total care is provided. At this writing she is fifty-seven years old. She seems terribly young to be so terribly, terribly ill.

I wonder about the distinctions we make regarding what is "normal" aging. These comparisons are dangerous. The distinctions have gotten us into trouble. We should never ignore the deteriorating mind; we should never accept it.

That we have done both has left some people thinking that progressive dementia is somehow acceptable for some individuals but not for others. I hear it all the time. Natural, maybe, for the old? Nonsense. There is nothing natural about it. There is nothing okay about it, and acceptance of this type of illness at any age allows us to make dreadful exceptions for all. The inherent social problems of living with dementia come from the absurd notion that confusion of this sort is a natural partner of aging and that therefore we must just live with it.

In the beginning of my mother's illness certain aspects of her behavior seemed acknowledgeable, familiar, normal. Among so many new and foreign actions they seemed somehow recognizable, although wrong. Wrong for her. Along with the hysteria and the psychotic delusions from which she suffered, there were actions based on simple forgetfulness. I had never before seen psychotic behavior such as hallucinations and accusations of family members. I had witnessed the repetitiveness associated with forgetfulness in the elderly, and knowing about this gave me something I could describe to the doctor in language I knew. The psychotic episodes just left me reeling.

My point is that even for me, who had so strenuously objected to the label of senility, the signs of that "senility" were new, and I reacted, in the beginning, as I would with a wholly incompetent person. I took away many of her functions. I overreacted. Certainly she should not be driving a car, but there was no reason that she should not be listened to, have her opinions sought, engage in topics of conversation other than her frustrating illness. Without accepting the word "senility," I had wholeheartedly accepted the misconception many people have that the old, or those behaving like the old, are incompetent and need to have everything done for them, and worse, that they have nothing to offer.

I was a mess until I got into a family support group and learned that there is a razor's fine edge between teaching helplessness and caring. I learned to prolong ability, not to rob freedom. I learned to utilize every shred of awareness she had and to supplement that which she had lost. Even now, in the nursing home, she is far from helpless.

The younger patient with Alzheimer's disease (AD) is terribly misunderstood right from the start. Two years before the diagnosis, when my mother's memory was bad but her determination to find a cure for her condition very strong, we went to every doctor we could think of. She readily agreed to a variety of tests and a remarkable range of treatments. She had a hysterectomy when it was suggested by one doctor that menopause might be the reason for her confusion. She went to a psychiatrist and two neurologists. She gave up alcohol. She engaged in more strenuous exercise. We even tried ginseng tea and megavitamin therapy. Her memory continued to decline.

As it became apparent that her memory problem was indeed progressive, a diagnosis was made. She was following the identifiable course of decline known as AD. Her life was being severely altered without her consent. She wanted the freedom to which she was so accustomed. She wanted to continue to be included in her circle of friends.

The friends presented a particularly difficult problem. They could not accept what was happening to her. It was easy to see that what she did and said looked and sounded so much like behavior their parents or grandparents had displayed that many just turned from her in haste. Many treated her as though she had brought this upon herself. Very few seemed able to accept her neediness. One woman in her fifties said to me that it was "just too strange to be seeing 'it' in someone my own age." She said that it "made her feel old."

The onset of her dementia frightened them. It seemed to be rushing death. One woman said that other illnesses such as cancer could not be helped, although some could be avoided, but "senility" was "supposed" to afflict the elderly and that this early onset threatened every one of my mother's contemporaries. It certainly seemed to. She had been born and raised in the small community in which she lived until she entered the nursing home. She knew everyone, and everyone knew her. She had many friends. Until she got sick.

My mother's age presented tremendous problems in terms of the cost of her care. Before she was diagnosed, she had to leave her job. The unspecified nature of her illness left her disability status open to interpretation, and eventually it was interpreted that she was not covered. She was too young for Medicare. The result was that by the time she was fifty-five years old both my father's and mother's life savings had been wiped out in caring for her. I always tell people that right after they get a diagnosis they should get a lawyer.

Many nursing homes are reluctant to take a young patient. Many families are reluctant to place a young patient. In my experience, age makes no difference to the patient by the time he or she is ready to be placed in a home. By virtue of her age and her earlier athletic activities, my mother is less frail than the other residents of the home. Before she entered the home, her strong, athletic nature presented a real problem to the attendants we had living with her. My mother was running them ragged. The agitation associated with the disease, combined with her physical strength, made her very difficult to contain safely. As a result, she was sedated. The medication caused her to appear far less able than she was in fact. The combination of the care provided by the attendants plus the medication left her totally restricted.

When she was placed in the home, her sedation was cut in half. She began to talk and smile again. She recognized my sister and me. She expressed herself more freely and appeared to be much happier. The nursing home, then, provided a less restricted environment. Before I saw her there, this was a very hard concept for me to understand. Many people had tried to convince me that she would be better off in a home. Some hinted that she would even "do" better. I never anticipated the dramatic benefit she was to derive from being in the home.

Perceptions and beliefs are hard things to alter. This disease takes swipes at everything we know about the family, about love, and about illness. My beliefs about health care and about freedom have been permanently altered. I am glad to have learned. I am glad that, having learned, I can provide the best alternative for my mother. She is not better because I have relinquished some of my beliefs about the young versus the old—but she is better off.

CHAPTER EIGHT

Caring for the Dementia Patient

Miriam K. Aronson, Ed.D.

DEALING WITH ALZHEIMER'S disease (AD) is not easy. It takes its toll emotionally, physically, socially, and financially. The family needs good information and a place to start. This chapter is intended as an overview of some of the more salient issues involved in caregiving.

General Guidelines for the Caregiver

1. *Obtain accurate information about AD.* You will need to learn about the symptoms, the course of the disease, and management and treatment options. This information will not only help you to know what to expect but will assist you in developing both short- and long-term plans. Information may be obtained from your family doctor or other helping professionals. It is also important to contact the Alzheimer's Disease and Related Disorders Association (ADRDA) at 1-800-621-0379 (Illinois: 1-312-853-3060) to locate a chapter near you

and to obtain some published materials and information about chapter services such as support groups.

2. *Maximize the patient's participation in planning for care.* The patient should be told as much as he or she wants to know or is able to understand about AD. Many patients are relieved to know they have a disease that explains their symptoms. Often, a response to being told is "Thank God I'm not going crazy." The patient should be told that his or her symptoms will likely get worse and should be encouraged to express his or her preferences for care. With whom does he or she want to live if the living arrangements must be changed? Would he or she want to participate in research about AD? Whom would he or she want to make medical decisions?

3. *Identify the person in charge (the primary caregiver).* It may be best to call a conference of members of the immediate family (spouse, children, siblings) to discuss the situation and begin to plan. An important outcome of a first meeting is to identify the person in charge. If there is an able spouse, he or she will usually assume the primary responsibility for care on a daily basis. However, it is important to ascertain whether this is realistic. For example, will a 90-pound wife be able to care for a 200-pound husband as he becomes more physically incapacitated? Or, even more fundamentally, what if the spouse is the primary breadwinner or must now go to work for financial survival? Can his or her salary cover the added cost of household help while he or she is working?

Can the burden of caring be shared? Are there other family members available to help on a daily basis? If adult children are unavailable on a daily basis, it is important for them to participate in the decision making and to assume some of the burden of dealing with administrative issues such as helping to assume financial control or to arrange for needed services, appointments, etc. It is most important that communication lines be kept open and that family members provide emotional support for one another.

4. *Reassess the living situation of the patient.* If he or she is living alone, the situation must be carefully evaluated. How is he or she managing? How *safe* is he or she? What is his or her geographic relation to the family? How much longer may he or she be able to remain alone? What are his or her preferences for future arrangements? For the patient who is residing with a spouse, is the situation appropriate to the condition of the patient? For example, if the patient is experiencing insomnia, is there room enough so that the well spouse can get needed sleep? Is there enough room in the house so that outside help can be employed? If changes are now necessary or will be necessary in the future, options should be explored. Consider the emotional, financial, and practical aspects of living arrangements. If possible, the patient should be moved as little as possible, since change may be disorienting for the already disoriented patient. See chapter 19 regarding services and chapters 15 and 16 regarding nursing-home placement.

5. *Set realistic goals.* The patient will become increasingly dependent, and his or her quality of life will be affected by the care received. The goals should be to maximize whatever function the patient has left. Use his or her strengths to provide opportunities for accomplishments and self-esteem. You undoubtedly will have to reorder plans and priorities. For example, projected future travel abroad should probably be rescheduled for now if the patient's impairment is mild and travel is feasible.

6. *Make realistic financial plans.* The family must explore the availability of benefits and entitlements, such as health insurance, disability insurance, Social Security disability, Medicaid, and other insurance. Additionally, they must figure out the best way to maximize available resources, remembering that the disease has a long course, during which the needs for care will escalate. Furthermore, the designation of who is to have financial control is important, as is the development of a strategy for the patient to relinquish this control. Entitlements are discussed in chapter 19 and legal/financial-planning strategies are contained in chapter 18.

7. *Identify a source of regular medical care and coordination.* During the long course of the illness, the patient will need medical supervision to maintain general health, treat whatever concurrent illness may develop, and prescribe medication for behavioral symptoms that may develop. The treating physician may assume responsibility for coordination of care; the family may consult with another health professional to provide coordination of care ("case management"); or one family member may assume the role of case manager, coordinating the care with the physician.

8. *Give the patient every opportunity to function at his or her maximum potential.* Activities should be planned that take the patient's level of ability into account. The disease impairs new learning, so enrollment in a course or a lecture series would not be appropriate. However, while the patient may not be able to learn to play a new piece of music, he or she may play a familiar piece very well. Whenever possible, substitutions or replacements should be made for lost function. For example, alternative transportation should be found for the patient who can no longer drive. Simplification should be practical: change the rules of the game to

correspond with changes in condition. At first the patient may be able to play bingo with letters and numbers, then numbers alone, then even fewer numbers.

9. *Do not make unrealistic demands on the patient.* As the
   disease progresses, it may cause a shortened attention
   span or a change in behavior and manners. The patient will not be able to participate in accustomed activities. For example, he or she may no longer be able
   to sit through an entire concert or show, but may enjoy the first hour or so and need to go home at inter-
   mission. The patient may not be able to understand a
   dramatic play or movie but may enjoy a tuneful musical or a familiar show. He or she may not be able to
   sit through a family holiday dinner and would best be
   involved in only a brief visit.

10. *Use outside services as required.* Homemaking help,
    transportation, patient-sitting services, day care, over-
    night respite, and a range of other needed services
    can be purchased and can significantly improve the
    quality of life for both patient and caregiver. And
    placement in a long-term-care facility should be con-
    sidered as a viable option. Martyrdom is not a healthy
    response. At-home help is discussed later in this
    chapter.

Becoming a caregiver involves assuming a whole new set
of responsibilities and roles. For some persons these changes
may require more adaptation than for others. Some persons
feel more comfortable in a take-charge position; others may
feel squeamish at first. Remember, adjustment is a gradual
process. As the disease progresses, routine daily activities
become more difficult. Interventions are suggested to prolong the patient's ability to care for himself or herself and,
where possible, to eliminate some of the more common
sources of danger. Following is some information about some
of the common symptoms and care issues.

Dressing, Bathing, Grooming

As with all aspects of caring for a demented person, activities of daily hygiene need to be simplified. Give the patient limited choices in getting dressed rather than presenting a full closet from which to select. For example, offer two shirts or dresses and let him or her choose one. One problem some caregivers face is the patient's insistence on wearing the same clothing day after day. Removing the articles of clothing at night, after the patient is asleep, may help eliminate this daily confrontation.

The patient may develop problems in dressing and undressing himself or herself. The important considerations are comfort and minimizing the amount of assistance required in getting the patient dressed. It can be helpful to replace shoes that lace with step-in shoes or sneakers with Velcro closings. Similarly, Velcro fasteners can be sewn to shirts and dresses to avoid the need for buttons. Pants and skirts with elastic waists are recommended, as they are easy to put on and front and back are interchangeable, removing another source of confusion. For women, the use of socks or knee-high stockings can replace panty hose. Choose easy-care clothes that are machine-washable, stain-resistant, and require no ironing.

At some point in the illness, Alzheimer victims may show an aversion to bathing and may become a difficult management problem for the caregiver. The resistance might be the result of confusion or an apparent fear of water. A few measures can be taken that may reassure the demented person as he or she bathes. Some spouses report that they can successfully bathe the patient by joining him or her in the shower. Some report getting better cooperation at one time of day over another. Still others have reduced the number of baths or showers per week, sponging the patient as needed in between. Grab bars attached to the wall can aid in getting the patient in and out of the tub, while a shower chair (a chair with holes in it so the water can drain) can provide a safe alternative for the unsteady patient. (Both items are available through surgical-supply stores or home-care catalogs.) Confused persons left unattended in the bath or shower may scald themselves when they are unable to regulate the water temperature. By lowering the temperature setting on the hot-water heater, such accidents can be avoided, and it is recommended that this be done early in the illness.

As the illness progresses, the caregiver of a demented patient may decide that it is no longer possible to maintain prior levels of grooming for the patient. Simplification of daily self-care tasks is the key. For women, a less elaborate hairstyle, such as a short haircut or permanent wave, can be helpful. The use of dry shampoo can ease any struggles caused while showering or bathing. A weekly appointment with a hairdresser who knows the patient and can handle her calmly is probably advisable. Makeup should be kept to a minimum. At a certain point in the disease it is no longer advisable for male patients to use razor blades; electric shavers are a much safer alternative if the patient remembers how to use one. Other patients may prefer a biweekly trip to the barber for a shave.

Nutrition: Eating and Feeding

There is no known nutritional cause or treatment for AD. Studies of lecithin (choline) supplementation have demonstrated little or no success in alleviating the memory loss or other cognitive symptoms of the disease. Deficiency diseases caused by low levels of vitamin B_{12} or folate, for example, may cause dementialike symptoms that may be alleviated by treatment, making a careful diagnostic evaluation very important (see chapters 2 and 4).

The nutritional status of the patient will have impact on his or her care and should be monitored throughout the course of the illness. The patient's optimal weight should be maintained. Obesity may pose difficulties for management of patients in terms of moving, bathing, and lifting. On the other hand, underweight and undernutrition may herald a coexisting illness or may contribute to debilitation. Weight loss may occur as a result of decreased food intake, markedly increased activity due to agitation, or depression. In addition, a substantial percentage of patients seem to experience an unexplained weight loss. Your physician should be contacted if there are noticeable significant and unexplained changes in weight or in food intake. Medical evaluation may be needed to investigate the causes of weight loss. Vitamins or high-calorie formula supplementation may be recommended for those patients whose intake is not adequate.

Food shopping, meal preparation, serving, and eventually feeding become responsibilities of the family caregiver. With time, certain adaptations will have to be made. For example, the caregiver will probably want to use less fragile dishes and linens and more substantial utensils. Mealtime schedules may require change. The patient may do better with smaller, more frequent meals. Mealtimes should be well structured and predictable. Additionally, eating is a social occasion, and conversation should be encouraged. The involvement of the patient in food activities is to be encouraged insofar as is practical. For example, the moderately impaired patient may be able to help with clearing the table or drying the dishes. When the patient becomes nonconversant, mealtime may become very lonely for the caregiver. Installation of a small television set, radio, or stereo in the dining area may make mealtimes more comfortable.

Through the course of the illness, food tastes may change. Some patients may develop a preference for sweets; others may tend to use salt excessively; still others may tend to eat inappropriately, for example, eating mayonnaise straight from the jar or butter from the dish. Caregivers may thus have to regulate dietary intake increasingly. They may need to hide foods they wish to limit and, in some instances, keep the refrigerator locked. Caregivers will need to handle all food activities, even such simple tasks as putting condiments on food or serving coffee with milk and perhaps sugar. Patients with multi-infarct dementia (MID) may require more dietary regimentation than those with AD, as control of blood pressure, diabetes, and cholesterol may be essential to controlling the risks for additional ministrokes.

Some patients will forget they have eaten almost immediately after a meal and will insist they are hungry. In some cases, distraction may work. (Let's go for a walk. How about a game of gin rummy?) In other cases, demands for food will persist. It is suggested that lower-calorie snacks such as vegetable sticks and fruit be offered at these times. For those patients who are almost constantly demanding food, items from meals such as dessert and bread may be used as snacks.

In the later stages, confusion and apraxia (the inability to carry out purposeful movements) may interfere with the ability to eat, and caregivers may focus on encouraging food intake rather than limiting it, as they may have done earlier on. It may be necessary to cut foods, to supply the appropriate utensil with each dish, or to eliminate the use of utensils. Finger foods such as sandwiches and cut-up fruits and vegetables may become necessary. Liquids may become easier for the patient to handle than solids. At this point, encouragement of more calories in less volume may be prudent, for example, cream soups versus broth; supplemental shakes. If the patient is placed in a nursing home, it is important for families to share information with dietary staff regarding the patient's food preferences and adaptations that have worked for him or her.

Care must be taken to see that the patient's intake of liquids is sufficient to avoid dehydration. Patients should be encouraged to drink six to eight glasses of liquids daily. Special attention to liquid intake must be paid if the patient has reduced his or her food intake during spells of fever and during hot weather.

Your dentist should examine the patient's teeth early in the course of the illness and perform the necessary dental treatment or repairs so that the patient can chew his or her food comfortably. Appliances such as bridges and dentures should be as simple as possible, as the patient will become increasingly unable to keep track of removable appliances. Furthermore, good oral hygiene in terms of brushing and food removal should be part of routine care. The dentist may have to work with both the patient and caregiver to assure at least minimal routine care.

When patients become unable to eat on their own or with reasonable assistance from their caregiver, basic decisions must be made regarding whether medical interventions for feeding such as insertion of a tube or other device are to be instituted. Care and treatment decisions are discussed in chapters 16 and 20.

Medications

The person with AD may be taking medications for the relief of related symptoms such as insomnia, depression, paranoia, agitation, and anxiety as well as for any other coexisting conditions. It is most important that the treating physicians know about *all* drugs that are being prescribed for a given patient. As memory deteriorates and confusion increases, certain steps should be taken to ensure the safe and proper use of these drugs. For a person in the early stages of dementia who lives alone, a schedule can be maintained with simple interventions such as unit dosing, use of longer-acting drugs to simplify the drug schedule, or arranging for administration of drugs by a family member, neighbor, or other responsible person.

As the disease progresses, it may become inadvisable for the dementia victim to administer his or her own medications. At this time, too, it is important that the home be "accident-proofed" in terms of the accessibility of drugs. All medications and other potentially toxic substances should be kept out of the reach of the confused person. Moreover, all unused medications should be discarded. Safety caps on medication bottles may provide additional prevention, since they may deter a demented person from getting a drug that is not intended for his or her use, but don't count on them.

As the impairments in function become more severe, the victim may no longer be willing or able to swallow a capsule or pill. At this point, alternate means of administration such as use of liquids or drug suspensions or crushing pills and serving them in a food such as applesauce may become necessary. The caregiver may seek instructions from the physician or the pharmacist regarding the availability of alternatives and how to work with them. Furthermore, as the disease progresses and the brain becomes more compromised, a patient's drug threshold may change. Often he or she may become sensitive to smaller doses, and previously established regimens may need reevaluation. Abrupt changes in level of confusion or behavior may be due to drug sensitivities. Additionally, changes such as increases in restlessness, changes in posture, or frequent occurrence of falls must be noted and reported to the physician. It is thus important for families to maintain close contact with the physician regarding the monitoring of drugs.

Caregivers should always check with the treating physician regarding the use of alcohol and nonprescription drugs. These may have potentially harmful side effects and interactions with prescription drugs.

"Taking Things Away"

There are several issues beyond those of personal care that must be faced by caregivers of demented patients. Some of the more difficult decisions to be faced involve the restriction of activities for the victim of AD.

Usually at a point relatively early in the disease, the patient begins to experience difficulty in handling finances, if that had previously been his or her responsibility. The checkbook may no longer balance, bills may go unpaid or be paid multiple times, and money may be lost or spent at a greater rate than is prudent. Alternatively, the patient may become inappropriately tight with money, refusing to pay any bills. The caregiver must take over financial management, perhaps for the first time in the relationship. While this may be difficult for both patient and caregiver to accept at first, it is a necessary step to which both caregiver and patient will adjust. Relinquishing financial control is a necessity, but many patients like the independent feeling of having cash in their pocket or pocketbook. Rather than taking away all cash from the patient who loses money, some families find it easier to give him or her defined amounts of money to maintain a sense of independence and consider the potentially lost money well spent. Set a limit, based on prior life-style. Some families may provide the patient with $10 or $20 at one time; others, $100 or more. Multiple single dollar bills will seem like more money than a few larger-denomination bills.

The conflict between maintaining a level of independence and ensuring safety often surfaces around the issue of the patient's traveling alone. Families of dementia victims too often wait until some calamity occurs that forces upon them the recognition of their loved one's deteriorating condition. Even the most routine excursions can become suddenly unfamiliar for the Alzheimer patient. Rather than continuing to allow the demented person to travel alone and risk getting lost, trips should be limited to local areas within walking distance. The patient should wear an identification bracelet at all times in the event that he or she does become lost.

The caregiver may choose to continue to have his or her patient run errands in order to provide a feeling of usefulness. Many times the demented person will let the caregiver know when he or she is beyond the point of being capable of performing apparently simple tasks. A trip to the bank, for example, may one day overwhelm the patient even though all the paperwork has been prepared by the caregiver and the route is a familiar one; he or she may feel better if a companion comes along on the errand. When a patient returns home in a frightened or bewildered state, with a routine chore not completed, it may be time to re-evaluate that person's competencies.

Driving is often another area of conflict between caregiver and Alzheimer patient. While some persons with AD are somewhat aware of their limitations and voluntarily give up complex tasks such as driving, many patients insist on driving long after their abilities are impaired. The caregiver in these cases must do whatever is necessary to keep the demented person from driving, not only for the patient's own safety but for that of other persons. Removal of car keys from the patient's possession is a difficult but important step. If this is not possible, removing the distributor cap or disconnecting the starter wire may be a temporary deterrent. Sometimes simple suggestions such as "I'll drive today and let you rest" may work. In other situations the caregiver may have to resort to confiscating the actual license and asking the family doctor to "prescribe" that the patient stop driving; or in rare cases, official action may have to be taken through the Bureau of Motor Vehicles, usually by requesting that the patient be retested. In some instances patients may be convinced to stop driving when they are told that the insurance company will not insure someone with their condition.

The problem of restricting the patient from driving may be especially acute when the well spouse does not drive. If this is the case, it is strongly urged that the well spouse think about taking driving lessons and getting a license. In one Alzheimer family, the wife got her license at age sixty-five.

In the case of a person living alone or with other family, alternate transportation must be provided so that the patient may retain a level of mobility and socialization. Provision of a charge account with a local taxi company may be a viable alternative, as may be an arrangement with a neighbor to provide transportation for a reasonable fee; or in those cases in which there is household help, it is preferable to hire a person who can drive.

Personality Change

A change in personality is a hallmark of AD. Eventually, the "person" residing in the body of the patient is not the original person. For this reason, a film about AD is entitled *Someone I Once Knew;* a recent book, *The Loss of Self.* The changes can be most pronounced, and the new behaviors of the person can be annoying, unpredictable, and embarrassing. A formerly powerful business tycoon, currently unable to make even the simplest decision, now asks his wife, "Can I sit in this chair?" "Should I eat the grape?" A former professor who was exceedingly polite and proper began to speak in four-letter words and was a constant source of embarrassment for his wife, who then decided to curtail his social involvements. A previously docile person may become agitated, and an extroverted, active person may become withdrawn. Agitation, hostility, and paranoia may develop. Sometimes flashes of the patient's real personality may reemerge, usually on a very fleeting basis, bewildering family members.

Family members often find these changes in personality very hard to deal with. They are, in fact, sources of protracted grieving. The original person has been lost, but not exactly. His or her mind is dying, but the body lives on. It's hard to remember that the person is not your loved one, but it helps if you can detach yourself enough to accept this.

Sexuality and Alzheimer's Disease

The need for affection and intimacy are basic human needs that persist well into the illness. Patients become anxious and uncertain and often cling to their spouses, relentlessly seeking constant companionship and reassurance. The patient may frequently repeat to the spouse how much he or she loves her or him. Despite these expressions of love, the ability of the patient to initiate lovemaking may be lost, although the capacity to respond remains intact. The need to initiate may be uncomfortable for a spouse who is unaccustomed to doing so. Some spouses report a continuing good sexual relationship until well into the middle course of the illness, while others report the loss of reciprocity early on. As with other aspects of the relationship, sexual experiences are very likely to be adversely affected by the illness.

In the early stages of the disease, males may become impotent, and this problem may contribute to their seeking medical advice. Sometimes, in relatively few cases, there may be a markedly increased libido that may be tiresome and annoying for the well spouse. Spouses report some success in dealing with increased libido with use of distraction; use of postponement—"later," "tomorrow," etc.; or in some situations, repeated refusal.

At times, the well sexual partner may feel a sense of revulsion, not having the same feelings for what remains of his or her original spouse. This may heighten the level of guilt and tension for the well spouse. As the spouse's dementia progresses and behavior becomes more regressive, distancing may occur even if the relationship was undisturbed earlier.

Misidentification of others—such as the patient's not

knowing who the spouse is—is a prominent feature of AD. It is especially painful for the caregiving spouse, to whom this misidentification may manifest itself as sexual rejection. One wife dismissed her husband from the bedroom, saying, "You're not my husband." When he tried to explain, she replied, "If you're Sam, you're Sam number one, and my husband is Sam number two." Misidentification is a disease symptom over which the patient has no control and not necessarily a conscious rejection, but it hurts nonetheless.

At some point in the illness it may become necessary for the well spouse to move out of the bedroom or vice versa for various reasons: The patient may not be sleeping at night, and the pacing and physical activity may be too disruptive or exhausting. The patient may be incontinent and may require frequent linen changes. The patient may have an around-the-clock attendant who stays in the room with him or her. The patient may develop peculiar sleep habits such as sleeping in a favorite chair or on a couch. This move may herald a change in the sexual relationship, as well.

Loosened Inhibitions

Loss of inhibitions and inappropriate sexual behavior are, in fact, relatively rare in AD and may perhaps be more commonly associated with related disorders such as Pick's disease. In AD, inappropriate sexual behaviors may be concomitants of the changes in personality that do occur. A very staid clergyman was discovered engaged in sexual acts with animals by his horrified family. A previously polite professor made sexually suggestive remarks to his granddaughters. These types of changes may be sources of tremendous embarrassment for families. Fortunately, explicitly bizarre sexual behavior is rare and usually occurs during a passing phase. As the patient becomes more regressed, masturbation may become more commonplace.

Questions relating to sexuality may arise throughout the course of the illness, and the caregiver may need to seek a physician's advice in dealing with them.

Sleeplessness

As the disease progresses, changes may occur in the sleep-wake cycle. Sometimes it is possible to structure the patient's time and environment to minimize the associated problems. Following are some suggestions:

- Arrange the patient's schedule so that day is differentiated from night in terms of getting dressed, stimulation, and activities and try to limit daytime sleep to a *brief* nap or two—no prolonged sleep.

- Set a realistic bedtime. Most adults require six to eight hours of sleep. Awakening at 4:00 A.M. may thus not represent any sleep problem for the patient who went to sleep at 8:00 P.M.

- Use a small night-light in the bedroom and bathroom to minimize confusion in case the patient awakens or needs to use the bathroom.

- Make sure the bed and bedroom are comfortable and familiar. The patient may enjoy a favorite photograph or other memento on his or her nightstand. The patient may prefer to use a favorite blanket or to wear specific nightclothes.

- Should the patient awaken during the night, try to remain calm and softspoken and encourage his or her return to sleep.

- Limit the patient's intake of liquids immediately before bedtime.

- Eliminate or limit caffeine in the patient's diet. Caffeine is present in coffee, tea, cola drinks, and chocolate.

- If the patient tends to wander at night, install an alarm on the outside door or a lock in an unlikely place (such as near the bottom of the door) to prevent the patient's leaving home. Doors to stairwells or other dangerous places should be locked or gated off to prevent accidents. Dangerous and potentially dangerous items should be removed from the reach of the confused wandering patient, for example, medications, scissors, knives, matches, car keys.

- Do not lay out the patient's clothing for the next day. This may be a confusing clue, and if he or she wakes up disoriented during the night, he or she may get dressed inappropriately.

- Encourage the patient to take a bath or a whirlpool bath before bedtime or during a period of insomnia. This may be soothing and relaxing and enable him or her to sleep.

- Soft music may be soothing and may be helpful at bedtime.

- Sometimes a glass of warm milk, decaffeinated or herbal tea, a glass of beer or wine, or a tepid bath before bedtime may be calming. You might also want to try giving the patient 1,500 mg. of tryptophan.

- Uncomfortable or painful conditions such as arthritis or leg cramps that may interfere with sleep should be treated by the physician.

Depression, which often accompanies AD, may cause sleep difficulties. Symptoms of depression may include crying, sadness, weight loss, slowing down, social withdrawal, and expressions of hopelessness and worthlessness. If your patient has these symptoms, you should discuss them with your physician, who may decide to prescribe antidepressant medication.

For those families with larger homes, hiring a night shift of help may be helpful. If the patient is tended to, the caregiver is able to rest. A nighttime aide could bathe the patient, take care of grooming—shaving, shampooing, nail cutting—go on walks with the patient, read to him or her, or listen to music with him or her.

If various environmental manipulations fail, it may be necessary to obtain a prescription from your physician for a tranquilizing or sedating drug. Drugs should be used for sleep as infrequently as possible, as their effectiveness may diminish with prolonged use. Furthermore, patients wake up confused while on these drugs. On the other hand, if the patient's sleeplessness is disrupting the entire household and the caregiver is not getting needed sleep, use of medication may be necessary in order to maintain the patient at home.

Wandering

Wandering is a common occurrence in AD. It may be a result of a person's becoming lost or disoriented, it may be aimless, or it may be an expression of restlessness.

A patient may feel lost when away from his or her familiar environment, when he or she goes on an errand and forgets in mid-errand where he or she is. Similarly, when a person moves to a new environment—a new home or a nursing home, or even when he or she begins a day-care program—he or she may become more disoriented, and wandering may be an expression of his or her determination to "go home." Unexplainable or aimless wandering may reflect boredom or a need for exercise. Sometimes wandering may conceivably be a catastrophic reaction—fleeing from the unfamiliar or unpleasant. Wandering may occur more frequently at night, when the patient may be more disoriented generally.

Management of wandering is a perplexing problem for caregivers in all settings. Not only do families have difficulty at home, but this symptom may make patients difficult or sometimes impossible for professional caregivers in other settings such as day-care facilities or nursing homes.

Here are a few general suggestions:

1. Every patient should always wear an identification bracelet with his or her name on one side and, on the other, an indication of his or her condition—"memory loss"—and a telephone number to be called in the event of a problem. This is more effective than an ID card in a wallet that may easily become separated from the patient. Bracelets may be individually obtained and engraved or ordered from a commercial service, which may be located through your pharmacy.

2. The house should be accident-proof. Keep medications and toxic substances such as cleaning agents out of reach and locked up so that they are inaccessible to the patient. Likewise, potentially hazardous items such as guns, knives, scissors, matches, razors, and power tools should be inaccessible to the wandering patient. Gate off stairs so that the confused, wandering patient cannot easily fall. Install locks in unfamiliar places—for example, at or near the bottom of the door. Unused exit doors and windows should be securely locked. Install a simple alarm on the front door so you'll be alerted to any unexpected attempts at leaving. It's wise to "disable" a gas stove at night, either by using the shut-off valve or removing the knobs, and to hide the car keys.

3. Medication may be prescribed by the patient's physician to attempt to control agitation and/or restlessness; however, it is conceivable that agitation may be a side effect of some medications. Thus, careful monitoring of the patient's symptoms and medications should be done.

4. Try to distract the wandering patient, who may, at times, agree to sit down for a cup of tea or to watch television or to listen to music.

5. There are physical restraints that can be used at home to keep a patient in a chair or a bed. The most common of these devices is a posey, which should be prescribed by the patient's physician and for the use of which the caregiver will need instruction, probably from a nurse. Sometimes it is practical to use a geriatric chair, which is a high-backed chair with a tray that serves both as a surface on which to eat, do crafts, or rest things and as a mechanism to keep the patient in the chair. This may be especially useful for the caregiver to use while he or she is in the bathroom, cooking, or otherwise unable to supervise the patient closely. A geriatric chair may be purchased from a surgical-supply store. Patients must not be immobilized continuously. The physician's instructions should indicate a schedule that includes movement and exercise.

6. Structuring environmental cues may be helpful sometimes in reducing wandering. For example, some patients may not go outside without their shoes or their coat, so keeping outerwear out of the patient's sight may be an effective deterrent.

7. In some cases, staying with the patient and reassuring him or her in a new environment—for example, during an acute hospitalization or for the first few days of a day-care program—may be soothing.

Some strategies may work at some times but not others. Wandering is a manifestation of impaired brain function, about which little is yet known. Caregivers must determine for themselves—often by trial and error—what works best for their patient.

Falling

Later in the course of dementia, patients may begin to fall frequently for no apparent reason. Researchers have indeed confirmed an association between mental impairment and falling but as yet have no scientific explanation. Meanwhile, it is important for caregivers to manipulate the environment to minimize the possibility of falling. Some suggested interventions follow:

1. Minimize obvious environmental hazards such as slippery floors, slippery bathtubs and showers, broken steps, and loose throw rugs.

2. Use good lighting to minimize confusing shadows and glare. Make sure the patient wears eyeglasses or a hearing aid, if necessary, so that he or she receives environmental cues.

3. Declutter the environment. It is more difficult for a confused person to navigate around an obstacle course. Less furniture and bric-a-brac are recommended. It is strongly urged, however, that familiar items be maintained.

4. Use of color may be effective in helping a patient decipher his or her environment. For example, painting the bathroom door a bright color may help the patient distinguish it from other rooms.

5. Have the patient wear safe footwear.

6. Make sure that the patient's clothing is not too long, making him or her vulnerable to tripping.

7. Install grab bars in the bathroom to enable the patient to hold on and stabilize his or her balance while using the tub, shower, and toilet.

8. Limit the patient's access to stairs if he or she is prone to falling. This is especially important regarding night wanderers, who may be increasingly confused while wandering.

9. Keep nonessential doors and windows locked to minimize the chance of accidents.

10. Limit the patient's outdoor exposure in bad weather. The patient may be unable to stay on a shoveled path or walk around an ice patch.

11. Make sure the patient gets adequate exercise to maintain strength and muscle tone.

12. If the patient suddenly starts to fall frequently, contact your physician, as this may be a side effect of medication or an indication of another illness.

Incontinence

Incontinence usually occurs later in the course of the illness. It presents an added burden and challenge for the caregiver, who must now deal with keeping the patient comfortable, minimizing embarrassment, and dealing with the increased amounts of laundry and bathing and skin-care needs that accompany this condition.

Fortunately, there are an assortment of adult undergarments and diapers available. Additionally, your physician or home-care nurse may recommend various techniques for dealing with this problem, such as anticipatory timing, catheters, enemas, etc.

It is important to note that incontinence usually occurs later in the illness. If a patient with early dementia suddenly starts to have "accidents," the difficulty may be related to a coexisting and potentially remediable illness or problem— possibly a urinary-tract infection. Do not assume incontinence is "normal" in an Alzheimer patient in the early stages of the illness.

Prior to the development of incontinence the patient may become increasingly unable to find the bathroom without assistance, to manage his or her clothing, and to maintain an acceptable level of personal hygiene. Thus, the development of incontinence will usually follow a gradual process of difficulty with toileting.

Incontinence may necessitate having the patient wear only easily laundered clothing. Moreover, the caregiver may be faced with increased amounts of soiled laundry, which may necessitate purchase of a home washer and dryer, if these are not easily accessible, or outside assistance with this chore. Medical management of incontinence is discussed in chapter 9.

Treatment Decisions

As the Alzheimer patient becomes increasingly impaired, he or she becomes more unable to participate in decision making regarding his or her own care. It is important, therefore, that early on in the illness the wishes of the patient and family regarding care and treatment be clarified.

All decisions should be based on several factors, including the patient's and family's values and beliefs, their preferences, their religion, and the implications for quality of life.

DESIGNATING A SURROGATE DECISION MAKER

The patient should be encouraged to designate one person—usually a family member—as a *surrogate decision maker*. The patient may sign a durable power of attorney for health care, a living will, or a variety of trust agreements. In some cases, more formal court proceedings, such as conservatorship or guardianship, may become necessary. Various decisions will be necessary during the course of the illness, and it is advisable to attempt to avoid court involvement where possible. The various options are reviewed in chapters 18 and 19.

ELECTIVE TREATMENTS

Careful consideration must be given to the performance of any elective diagnostic or surgical procedures. Generally, hospitalization and anesthesia should be avoided or minimized whenever possible, as they will be disorienting (at least temporarily) and possibly debilitating. If elective procedures can be anticipated, they should be done as early in the dementing illness as possible. For example, if cataract surgery is necessary, its chances for success diminish with the increasing cognitive impairment of the patient. Dental procedures may have to exclude the purely cosmetic.

PARTICIPATION IN RESEARCH

Early on it is important to ascertain the patient's views regarding participation in research protocols. Does the patient want to try an experimental treatment, and if so, what type of procedures would be acceptable? For example, would the patient submit to neurosurgery for a brain biopsy or for implantation of a technological device, such as a pump for delivery of medication? Would the patient agree to a spinal tap (lumbar puncture) for research purposes? Would the patient take medication?

TREATMENT SETTING

If possible, family members should attempt to determine from the patient some indication of his or her preferences regarding where and how he or she wishes to be treated. Some patients will state clearly, "I do not wish to be a burden to my children and want to be put in a home when I get bad." Others may say, "I want you to promise that you would never put me away." Family members should avoid making promises they may not be able to keep. "Never" is a long time. Circumstances may change, and ill-conceived promises may become impossible to keep. Patients with dementia will be able to live alone only for a limited period and will need to move to a more structured, supervised environment. For patients who have no available family caregivers, placement in a nursing home may be a necessary intervention. And for those patients whose care needs exceed the capabilities of their family caregivers, placement in a nursing home may be a positive intervention.

TERMINAL-CARE ISSUES

Patients in the end stage of the disease may be unable to obtain adequate nutrition via oral feeding. The family must decide what purpose nutritional heroics—for example, tube feedings, surgery—would serve. If they conclude that this intervention would merely prolong the process of dying, they must determine whether this would be appropriate care. Furthermore, family members must ascertain how much they wish to pursue treatment of other illness—for example, administration of antibiotics for pneumonia in the comatose, vegetative end-stage patient. The family must develop a clear decision regarding whether the terminal patient should be resuscitated if his or her heart stops. If there is written material by the patient or a document such as a living will, the decision should be based on this. If there are no documents available and if there is no officially designated guardian, the family should make the needed decisions and clearly communicate their wishes to the physician involved. Terminal-care issues are discussed in detail in chapter 20.

A caregiver who maintains a patient at home may have decided against any heroics; however, as the patient becomes more terminal, "panic" may set in, and the caregiver may be tempted to call the rescue squad. This action may serve to negate an earlier decision. One wife did this when her husband had a seizure but then realized the implications of her reaction and declined to allow the ambulance to remove her husband to the hospital, since they had both wanted him to die at home.

Autopsy serves as a measure of diagnostic certainty for families while simultaneously providing needed tissue for AD research. Whether an autopsy will be performed can and should be decided well in advance. This information and the necessary instructions from the pathologist should be communicated to the physician. Each ADRDA chapter has an Autopsy Network representative who can be helpful in providing information and in making arrangements.

Caring for Yourself, the Caregiver

You, the caregiver, may be so involved in caring for your loved one that you are tempted to forget about yourself. It is strongly recommended that you include yourself in your caregiving plans. Listen to your body; get adequate rest and sleep. Take your medications as prescribed. Get regular medical care and try to keep your level of stress as low as possible. Here are some more specific suggestions.

1. *Begin to let go.* AD is an affliction over which neither you nor the patient has control. You, as the caregiver, must learn to put some emotional distance between the patient and yourself. You must recognize that as the patient's dependency increases with advancing disease, your needs for independence will increase. Thus, with time, your needs and those of the patient will diverge, and adjustments will have to be made. You will find that caregiving is not only a means of achieving an unparalleled closeness but also, of necessity, a gradual process of letting go. As the person

you knew slips away from you, so must you begin to let go and concentrate on your own emerging needs.

2. *Work on resolution.* You cannot erase the past history of your relationships. Try to work toward a sense of closure and to resolve conflicts rather than to create new ones. Dementia may make good relationships less good and bad relationships worse. It may be difficult for you to control your anger, and you may impulsively want to say some things that may make you feel guilty later. Remember, you cannot "take back" things you didn't mean to say, so it's best to ventilate away from the patient.

3. *Avoid martyrdom.* Martyrdom may lead to isolation, which, in fact, may create more stress. Caring for a patient with AD is a big job. Seek and accept whatever help you can get. Friends and relatives often do not know how to help. You have to ask them specifically for what you need. You may have to purchase outside services as the patient's care needs increase.

4. *Use a confidant.* Share your feelings and experiences with someone you trust. This may be a family member, a friend, a neighbor, a member of the clergy, or a medical or mental-health professional. You might attend a support group, as well. The confidants you use may be different at different times and in different situations.

5. *Look for the silver lining in the black cloud.* While everything may seem bleak at this point, remember that no one goes unchanged from the impact of AD. You will be forced to do things you never knew you were capable of doing and probably will grow as a result of the experience. In the course of dealing with AD, spouses have learned to handle complex financial investments, to drive a car, to step in and run a business, to travel independently.

6. *Listen to your own feelings.* If you are very tired, you probably need to slow down and rest. If you're feeling ill, you may need medical attention yourself. If you are feeling sad or blue, no wonder; however, if you are crying much of the time, not sleeping, losing weight, and have difficulty getting through your normal routine, you may possibly have a clinical depression that may require treatment and should discuss these symptoms with your family physician.

7. *Attend a support group.* Attendance at a support group may provide information, the opportunity to give and get practical caregiving tips and emotional support, and the chance to think about rebuilding your own social supports and to plan for the future. The nearest chapter of ADRDA can help you locate a support group.

8. *Use respite services.* Every caregiver needs time away from caregiving responsibilities, whether an hour at a time, an afternoon or evening at a time, a day at a time, a weekend, or a week away. You must seek out opportunities to get this relief whether from family, friends, paid workers, community agencies, or a combination. The local ADRDA chapter may have its own respite program or may maintain a list of community resources.

9. *Ventilate.* Express your frustrations, but away from the patient as much as possible. At times you may find yourself screaming at the patient to no avail. He or she does not mean to be that way. He or she will forget what happened, but you will wind up feeling guilty. It is better to find some other outlet for release. You may do this verbally, talking with a confidant or counselor or in a support group. Or you may find physical exercise a great source of relief. Take a brisk walk, attend a dance class or an exercise class, swim, work out in a gym, or play a sport such as tennis or golf.

10. *Be good to yourself.* One of the things you may miss the most is positive feedback from the patient. Not only are thank-yous gone, but so, too, are birthday and holiday celebrations and gifts. So be good to yourself—go to the barber or beauty shop; eat at a restaurant with friends; see a movie; buy a new item of clothing; buy something decorative for the house. You *deserve* it!

11. *Take things in manageable chunks.* While you need to plan and make decisions, not all decisions have to be made at one time. Sometimes it may be best to try to get a little distance before doing anything dramatic. It is best to take things in discrete portions—a day at a time, a week, a month, a year. You may not initially be able to deal with too much "down the road." Sometimes it may feel like a big accomplishment just to get through a bad day.

Using Outside Help

At some point it may become necessary for the caregiver to employ outside help in the home. The point at which the caregiver will acknowledge the need for additional help will vary for different caregivers. For some, it may be when the patient is very agitated; for others, it may be when the patient becomes incontinent; for still others, it may be not until the patient becomes bedbound. Not only will the trigger of need be different but also the circumstances. Some persons may live in close quarters and find having help in the house an intrusion, while others may welcome the assistance and companionship. Some may feel somehow inadequate because they can no longer go it alone.

WHERE TO START

1. *Try to define what help you need.* If the patient lives alone, companionship/supervision may be required earlier in the course than if family members are present. For example, if the patient is manageable during the day but up all night, perhaps a night shift of help would be appropriate. Perhaps a live-in person who would come in for five and a half days per week would be appropriate when family members are employed. What are the hours you would ideally like to have help? If the patient is still in the same bedroom with the spouse, sleeping accommodations may have to change, so that the helper can tend the ill spouse while the well spouse sleeps.

2. *Estimate the cost and identify potential sources of payment.* Will the shifts be eight or twelve or twenty-four hours? Is the rate of pay hourly or a fixed fee? Is the patient entitled to Medicaid? What cost-sharing or reduced-fee programs are available in your community?

3. *Write a job description.* What are the aide's duties? Is there other help (e.g., cleaning, driving)? To whom will the helper be directly responsible—you, the caregiver or an adult child? Is the aide expected to wear a uniform? Is the aide expected to travel if the family travels (e.g., to a country home)? Will the person be expected to drive a car?

4. *Make the terms clear.*

    Schedule: What are the aide's hours? What are the patient's mealtimes? Will the aide eat with the patient? If not, when and where?

    Finances: If the aide takes the patient out for lunch or dinner or recreation, how is payment to be arranged?

    Compensation: What is the salary? Who pays agency fee(s)? For what services will extra pay be available—

for example, if the caregiver goes on vacation and twenty-four-hour coverage is required? Is carfare to be reimbursed? Is use of a car provided? If so, for what? What meals are provided? Are there any benefits—vacation days, sick days, insurance? What are the restrictions concerning the aide's use of the telephone?

QUALIFICATIONS

Special requirements: What special qualifications (or licenses) should this person have? For example, few insurance policies may pay for home care if provided by licensed personnel. Do you require special training or experience?

Language: Is the person English-speaking, or do you require another language because the patient has regressed to it?

Size: If the patient is large and requires lifting, the helping person needs to have the size and stamina to perform this duty.

Temperament: Is the patient paranoid? He or she would then likely respond best to a laid-back individual. If the patient is withdrawn, a more enthusiastic person may be effective.

Gender: Some families may prefer a male aide for a male patient.

Physical agility: If the patient is physically active and a wanderer, the helping person must have the physical stamina to keep pace.

SOURCES OF HELP—WHERE TO START?

It may not be easy. You may have to try more than one person or source until you find the right person.

Friends, family, and neighbors may be available to help or may be able to locate suitable candidates through word of mouth or to help with calling agencies and advertising.

Your local ADRDA chapter may maintain lists of resources.

Senior citizen centers often maintain lists of persons seeking employment. Members of support groups may help each other, perhaps helping to care for an additional patient during an emergency.

Home care agencies or nursing agencies can usually supply help on very short notice.

Other employment agencies—for example, the State Employment Service—may provide suitable candidates.

Students may be appropriate to fill in at times.

"Help Wanted" advertisements in the local paper are another source of supply.

Your case manager may be a good resource.

Your family doctor may have leads.

HOW MUCH HELP?

How much help is needed depends on the stamina of the primary caregiver, the availability of help from family and friends, what other services—such as day care—are utilized, and the family budget. Remember, time away for the caregiver is a necessity, and expenditure of funds for this purpose will be money well spent.

If maintaining help at home becomes logistically too cumbersome or too expensive, then placement of the patient in a residential care facility may become a more realistic alternative.

In summary, dealing with AD is a long process that requires significant amounts of thought and energy. No affected family goes unscathed; throughout this long process, however, family members may exhibit strengths and develop skills they never thought they had.

CHAPTER NINE

Treatment of Behavioral and Mood Changes

Lissy F. Jarvik, M.D., Ph.D., and David W. Trader, M.D.

AS WE AWAIT THE RESULTS OF research aimed at learning the cause(s) and finding ways to prevent Alzheimer's disease (AD) and related dementias, a systematic approach to symptomatic treatments can help us deliver comprehensive and humane care. In this chapter we will discuss some of the more common behavioral and mood changes of the Alzheimer patient as well as treatment and coping strategies that may help ease the burden on the families. The unique circumstances of each patient and each family must be taken into account in selecting treatment strategies. No strategy will

This work was supported in part by National Institute of Mental Health research and training grants (MH 36205, MH 40059, MH 17251) and the Veterans Administration. The opinions expressed are those of the authors and not necessarily those of the Veterans Administration.

be successful for all patients or at all times for any patient. Therefore, the patient's physician is expected to prescribe medications thoughtfully and to monitor them carefully.

Acknowledging Symptoms

In the early years of the illness, symptoms may go unnoticed, especially if the victim lives alone. Difficulties are often exposed when the person is faced with a novel situation or at times of crisis. The patient's reaction may be to try and conceal the difficulties because of the embarrassment a "mental problem" represents or the fear that the specter of "losing one's mind" arouses. Caregivers, too, may go through their own denial of problems. A caregiver can help the patient by acknowledging that there is something wrong and offering support. The person may be relieved to know that someone understands. Too often, however, intervention may be met with denial and resistance. For example, a spouse may be told, "There is nothing wrong with me—if you just keep my dinner hot instead of letting it get cold, I won't lose my temper." In that case, the wife might mention to her husband the next morning that he seems to be bothered by a lot of things these days. He may or may not agree. If he does not, she may have to wait until he indicates he needs help or until a crisis develops that brings the problem to everyone's attention. If the impaired person's behavior becomes socially unacceptable, hostile, or assaultive, providing that help may be difficult.

Forgetting

Prominent forgetfulness or memory loss is the hallmark of AD. It appears early in the course of the illness and is central to current diagnostic criteria.

Neither patient nor family members may recognize the seriousness of the problem. They may ascribe the difficulties to some other illness, a change in the work situation, or some other external event.

Mrs. C., a legal secretary, attributed her forgetfulness to lack of stimulation ensuing from forced retirement. She had worked for the same law firm for twenty-seven years. Despite her increasing slowness and decreasing productivity, no one wanted to fire her. When the firm switched from typewriters to word processors, however, Mrs. C. could not learn the necessary new skills and was therefore forced to retire.

Other patients accept their deficits and respond with appropriate coping mechanisms. Memory aids may help, especially early in the course of the illness. A calendar large enough to log daily activities is often useful so the patient can mark off days as they pass. For those patients who can understand what they read, it is important to compile a list of instructions to follow under various circumstances. A booklet containing names and frequently called numbers is often helpful. Sometimes pictures and familiar objects serve as memory aids. Sometimes it is helpful to label objects around the house, such as clothes, drawers, radio, television, walkers.

It should be stressed that *some forgetfulness is normal.* However, *severe memory loss is not part of the normal aging process.* The term "benign senescent forgetfulness" was introduced to differentiate normal age-related memory changes from "malignant senescent forgetfulness." The latter is characteristic of a progressive memory loss such as that seen in AD. In the benign form, now also called "age-associated memory impairment," a person has difficulty remembering relatively unimportant facts or parts of an experience (such as name, date, or place) but can recall the forgotten material at a later time. Clinicians use a variety of brief mental-status questionnaires to measure memory loss and to track the progress of the dementia. These include the Blessed Information-Memory-Concentration Test, the Ten-Item Mental Status Questionnaire, and the Mini-Mental State Examination. Depression may cause difficulties with concentration, which may resemble memory deficits.

Identification of memory deficits is crucial in developing management strategies. Information from the patient, family members, and other caregivers provides the basis for cognitive assessment. In addition, formal neuropsychological testing, stressing learning as well as remembering, may help determine whether a patient's forgetfulness is most likely due to dementia, depression, or normal aging.

Dementia patients may forget what is said to them, often within minutes, and following complex instructions becomes increasingly difficult.

> Prior to going to work, Mrs. G. asked her mother to prepare the pot roast, vegetables, and dessert for dinner that evening. Upon returning home, Mrs. G. found that nothing had been prepared. She became extremely angry at her mother, not realizing that her mother had been unable to remember the instructions long enough to carry them out.

Patients may forget appointments and important dates or neglect to relay important telephone messages. Sometimes patients themselves are the first to recognize that they have a memory deficit. Memory impairment affects most activities of daily living, activities that are taken for granted by those without memory problems. Patients may forget to turn off the stove; they may forget when they last ate and refuse to eat or eat too much. Patients may think that they have recently bathed when it may have been a week since their last bath.

Eventually, patients no longer understand time relationships. When asked for the date, they sometimes respond, "Oh, I don't have to pay attention to that anymore." They may be able to tell time from a watch but have no understanding of what 10:45 means. Also, if left alone, some Alzheimer patients think that they have been left for a longer time than is actually the case.

In the early phase of the illness, patients may have a better recollection of events that occurred years ago than of those of the previous week. Their ability to recall childhood events often gives the false impression that their memory is good. Even as the disease progresses, relatives may be unaware of the seriousness of the patient's impairment.

> Mrs. O. became increasingly despondent as her husband started calling her Katie, which was his first wife's name. On several occasions he told her to get out of the bed they shared. After all, they had been divorced, and she did not belong there.

Strategies

Recommendations designed to maintain higher intellectual functions as long as possible are based on clinical experience. Patients are encouraged to participate in tasks that keep them mentally and physically active. Clinical experience also teaches us that it is important to try to understand the patient's situation. Imagine being unable to tell time or not knowing how to ascertain the correct date or how to find your way home or even recognize your own home. Sometimes it helps to provide reassurance that you will not abandon the patient and to make it clear that you want to help.

Maintaining a routine schedule of activities along with structuring the environment is the foundation of the treatment of behavioral disorders. It tends to reduce the anxiety centered around forgetting and being lost.

The search for a drug or drugs effective in treating or improving memory has evolved considerably with our understanding of the physiology of the illness. At this time, however, there is no drug available that will retard the cognitive symptoms of the disease. An extensive discussion of drug-treatment strategies is contained in chapter 4.

Language Dysfunction

There are language changes that may follow a specific pattern in AD. Aphasia (e.g., errors of grammar and word choice) has been shown to be a persistent feature of AD. The language of Alzheimer patients is often free flowing but of an empty quality, with indefinite references (e.g., thing, it, they). Patients gradually lose the ability to find the right word (called anomia), usually starting with words they use infrequently. They may substitute descriptions for specific words. In wanting to use the word "purse," a patient may say, "I can't find my . . . you know . . . the thing I carry my money in." They may also substitute other words or syllables for the right ones (called paraphasias). For example, a patient may use the word "lurse" instead of "purse." Comprehension of both spoken and written language is also progressively impaired in AD. Patients may be able to read aloud, but they may not understand what they have read. In the terminal phases of AD, speech may be reduced to repetitive sounds.

It can be frustrating for the patient as well as the family to be unable to communicate properly. Unfortunately, there is no specific treatment for the language deterioration in AD. If a patient is having difficulty finding the correct word or expressing an idea, caregivers may reduce the stress by supplying the word or idea. Little is gained by having the patient struggle with this handicap.

Sleep Disturbance

Combined with their time disorientation, sleep disturbance in Alzheimer patients often results in night restlessness or insomnia. As research data are lacking concerning the treatment of insomnia in AD, the treatment recommendations are based on clinical experience; they are discussed by other authors (see chapter 8).

PHARMACOLOGICAL TREATMENT

If environmental measures are ineffective, then you may want to consider using medications. When given an hour or two before bedtime, they often relieve the early insomnia associated with dementia. One must be cautious, however, about the type of sleeping medicine used. Your physician will evaluate the situation and prescribe accordingly. Medications that are longer acting, such as flurazepam (Dalmane) and diazepam (Valium), have a tendency to stay active for many hours in the body. Short-acting drugs tend to produce high levels that drop off sharply, so that untoward effects may result from both extremes. These include symptoms of withdrawal such as shaking, sweating, tremors, and high blood pressure. Therefore, drugs with intermediate duration of action are desirable, such as chloral hydrate (500–1,000 mg.) and some of the drugs in the benzodiazepine family, such as lorazepam (0.25–0.5 mg.), temazepam (15–30 mg.), or oxazepam (10–15 mg.). These agents may be given either on an as-needed basis or at a regularly scheduled time. Benzodiazepines must be used with caution, as they may worsen cognitive deficits and can cause confusion, depression, agitation, and unsteady gait. Moreover, they may lose their effectiveness after a month of continued use. It is generally best to avoid barbiturates (e.g., secobarbital). Drugs should be reevaluated after one week and stopped, if possible, to avoid habituation or dependence.

Anxiety/Agitation/Assaultiveness

Anxiety, agitation, and assaultive behaviors associated with AD may manifest themselves in various ways, including pacing, fidgeting, yelling, throwing objects, refusing help, or hitting. Exact reasons for these behaviors are uncertain. Sometimes they may be secondary to tension, to feelings of loss or depression, to changes within the brain itself, to other physical illness, to pain, or to the side effects of medications. Assaultive behavior may occur even in persons who never demonstrated it in the past and may not be under the patient's control.

Reassurance and calm comforting may be sufficient to contain these disturbances. It is important, however, to try and understand possible reasons for the behavior. Is the patient frustrated about losing his or her memory? Or afraid of being abandoned? Is the home situation chaotic for other reasons? Most of the time there will be no obvious reason. Sometimes a person may need an object on which to focus the excess energy.

Mr. K. became frustrated with his wife, who would repeatedly take out and put in her dentures when going to bed at night. One night she fell asleep with her clothes on, and he noticed her playing with her necklace while asleep. From that time on he made sure she wore the necklace to bed, and she rarely replaced her dentures after that.

PHARMACOLOGICAL TREATMENT

Certainly not all anxiety is managed so easily, and medications may have to be employed when environmental changes are ineffective. Two general classes of drugs are frequently used for this purpose, benzodiazepines and neuroleptics. Although there are numerous reports of beneficial results, the research is limited and inconclusive for the use of these agents in the demented elderly.

Drugs in the benzodiazepine family, often called anxiolytics, were discussed in the previous section. The same strategy of using relatively short-acting agents in low doses applies here. One member of this class not mentioned previously is alprazolam. It has become one of the most popular drugs prescribed for the treatment of anxiety. Again, caution is needed in the demented elderly. They may have increased sensitivity to this type of medication, such that even low doses may cause problems. For example, these drugs may cause an increase in agitation that can be misinterpreted as a worsening of symptoms associated with the dementia, which may prompt the physician to mistakenly increase rather than decrease the dose. An alternative to the benzodiazepines in treating symptoms of anxiety can be a sedative antidepressant such as trazodone.

Neuroleptic medications (major tranquilizers, antipsychotics) are widely used and may be appropriate for those patients who respond adversely to other drugs, those who do not respond at all and are very agitated, and those who are psychotic. (The last condition will be discussed in the following section.)

The choice of a particular drug is based on avoiding adverse side effects, the most common of which are anticholinergic symptoms, extrapyramidal symptoms, a drop in blood pressure when standing up (orthostatic hypotension), and sedation. Anticholinergic side effects include dry mouth, blurred vision, constipation, difficulty urinating and urinary retention in the bladder (especially in men when there is an enlarged prostate gland), tremors, worsening of narrow-angle glaucoma, and at higher doses, confusion, hallucinations, and agitation.

Extrapyramidal symptoms include muscle rigidity, slowness, tremor, drooling, shuffling gait, and muscle spasms. Patients are sometimes unable to sit still (akathisia). This symptom may be confused with increased agitation due to the illness, and a physician may mistakenly prescribe more, rather than less, neuroleptic. Tardive dyskinesia is another risk of neuroleptic treatment, especially when used long-term. This condition is characterized by involuntary movements of the lips, tongue, and face.

The stronger neuroleptics (such as haloperidol and thio-
thixene), effective in small doses, have significant extrapyramidal side effects but produce less sedation and relatively
fewer anticholinergic side effects. The weaker neuroleptics
(such as chlorpromazine and thioridazine) cause more sedation, hypotension, and anticholinergic effects but fewer
extrapyramidal reactions than do the stronger compounds.

As is true of most medications, neuroleptics should be
given in smaller doses to older persons. Common starting
doses are 0.5–2 mg. haloperidol or 10–25 mg. thioridazine.
The dose is gradually increased, if necessary, depending on
side effects. When starting a neuroleptic, the physician must
clearly define the target symptoms to the caregiver so as to
avoid prolonged or unnecessary use. Clinical experience indicates that demented patients often benefit from neuroleptics. However, they should be prescribed with careful
attention to both the therapeutic and toxic effects. You should
keep in close contact with the patient's physician and advise
him or her of any suspected adverse reactions.

Suspiciousness/Hallucinations/Delusions

Alzheimer victims may become suspicious (or paranoid); they
may worry that someone is stealing from them or intends to
harm them. They may hide possessions and, when unable
to find them, accuse others of having stolen from them. They
may accuse the spouse of being unfaithful, as did the patient described by Alois Alzheimer in his original report on
the disease that now bears his name.

Patients may also develop visual or auditory hallucinations in which they see objects or hear voices that are not
apparent to anyone else. Sometimes delusions develop. These
are false personal beliefs that are firmly sustained despite
evidence to the contrary. For example, some demented patients may believe that their parents are still living when in

fact they are not, or they may believe that a spouse is someone else.

The first step in management is to have a complete medical and neuropsychiatric examination, since these symptoms, even in the patient with AD, may derive from a
coexisting medical illness or from side effects of medication.
Patients with hearing and visual impairments may be at increased risk for developing hallucinations and paranoid
symptoms.

Generally, assuring the patient that you are there for him
or her may be helpful. It is usually useless to try to argue
patients out of their false beliefs. Clinical experience indicates that neuroleptic drugs (as discussed in the previous
section) are effective in demented patients with hallucinations, delusions, or paranoid ideas.

Depression

Depression is one of the most common mood disturbances
associated with AD. What little literature there is suggests
that 15 to 55 percent of demented patients have concurrent
depression. This wide range reflects the differences in the
studies and also the difficulty of studying depression coexisting with dementia. The symptoms of depression include
impaired concentration and memory loss, apathy, slowness
of motor function, fatigue, sleep disturbance, and expressions of wanting to die. They may be difficult to recognize
in the demented patient, since they resemble those of the
dementia itself. Complicating matters further is the fact that
depressive illness may present as a dementia syndrome. That
is, depressive illness, especially in the elderly, can produce
memory, intellectual, and behavioral impairment that may
disappear upon appropriate treatment but may otherwise be
indistinguishable from a dementia due to degenerative brain
disease. This condition has been termed "depressive pseu-
dodementia," or the "dementia syndrome of depression."

Even though it is understandable that anyone suffering from so devastating an illness as AD would be depressed, not all patients are. Indeed, it is uncertain how much depression is related to the underlying brain damage, how much is a reaction to the loss of cognitive abilities, and how much is a combination of both.

Since there are specific treatments for depression but not for AD, we tend to treat depressive symptoms whenever they appear. Early in the illness a patient may do well with individual or group therapy, and psychotherapy has the advantage of lacking the side effects of drug treatment. On the other hand, there are disadvantages, including high initial cost (especially for individual psychotherapy) and scarcity of therapists.

PHARMACOLOGICAL TREATMENT

Antidepressant medications are widely used. Unfortunately, there is little research on the efficacy of antidepressants in depressed demented patients. Much of our knowledge has come from clinical experience and drug trials on depressed nondemented patients. The most common side effects involve anticholinergic properties of the tricyclic antidepressants, the drugs generally used first. These effects have been discussed earlier.

In prescribing antidepressants, the general rule is to start with low doses and increase them slowly. There is no clear consensus as to the preferred antidepressant drug. We generally start with nortriptyline (10 mg.), desipramine (25 mg.), trazodone (25 mg.), or doxepin (25 mg.) and avoid amitriptyline and imipramine. If there is no substantial improvement, the dose may be doubled after five to ten days. For some patients that is enough; others need higher doses. If initial treatment is unsuccessful with the first agent, another antidepressant is usually tried. Aside from the drugs mentioned above, monoamine oxidase inhibitors, such as phenelzine (15 mg.) are used. These drugs do cause orthostatic hypotension and also require a strictly controlled diet and a careful check of all medications that may cause a sudden rise in blood pressure (including decongestants and nose drops). Thus, they are generally used only where there is a reliable caregiver.

If drugs do not work and the patient is severely depressed (refuses to eat or is suicidal), then electroconvulsive therapy (ECT), or "shock treatment," is another option. Data are lacking on the efficacy of ECT in depressed demented individuals, but clinicians have seen patients improve on numerous occasions. ECT may be more effective and produce fewer side effects than medications.

Wandering

Wandering is a common behavior in Alzheimer patients and one of the most difficult problems to manage. Not only is the behavior unpredictable, causing caregivers to be constantly on guard, but patients may be endangered when they wander. Wandering may result from restlessness and pacing, or getting lost, or may occur with a change in environment. The patient may get lost in familiar or unfamiliar surroundings. Many strategies have been tried in dealing with the wandering patient. In general, structuring the environment can be helpful. Suggested strategies are discussed in chapter 8.

Family members often ask: "Is there any medication that can stop the wandering?" Presently, the answer is no. However, there are drugs that may reduce the restlessness and agitation, thereby improving comfort and daily functioning.

As a last resort, restraints may be used under supervision and with caution, even though they may increase agitation. While it is often distressing for the caregiver to have to restrain a loved one, there may be no other way to prevent injury. This is particularly true when the caregiver has to leave the room to prepare a meal, go to the bathroom, or just take a free moment. More acceptable than the usual re-straints may be a geriatric chair, a padded high-backed chair with a waist-level tray that serves as an activity surface as well as a means of preventing the patient from getting out of the chair.

Apraxia

During the course of AD, patients may lose the ability to carry out purposeful movements. This is known as apraxia. The patient may know what to do but is unable to do it. For example, in testing for such a problem, the examiner might ask the patient to tie shoelaces, wave good-bye, or button a shirt. As the illness progresses, the patient may walk un-steadily and have difficulty eating with utensils, undressing, bathing, or writing. It is sometimes difficult, however, to determine whether the patient cannot complete the task due to an inability to understand what it is or an inability to make the muscles work.

Apraxias usually appear after memory and language dis-turbances have become prominent. Their exact cause re-mains a mystery. There is no specific pharmacological treatment for these conditions. Caregivers can compensate for these deficits by assisting the patient with activities such as dressing or cutting the patient's food before it is served.

Incontinence

Incontinence, or the inability to control urine or bowel elim-ination, usually occurs late in the course of AD. Certainly either form can embarrass patients, disgust caregivers, and add to the caregiver's sense of burden. Most of our knowl-edge of incontinence accompanying dementia has come from clinical experience, as there are few scientific data.

The first step in treatment is a careful assessment by the

physician. For urinary incontinence, a complete history and physical examination, urinalysis, urine culture, and urine-residual-volume test will help identify most treatable conditions. Most causes of sudden onset of urinary incontinence are treatable and include infection, drug side effects, and obstruction. The most common cause of chronic urinary incontinence is an uninhibited neurogenic bladder, a condition causing patients to be unaware of the need to void and to inhibit spontaneous bladder contractions. If clinical evaluation does not identify another cause, treating the patient for presumed neurogenic bladder may help.

Frequent toileting is, therefore, the initial treatment of choice. It may be useful for the caregiver to maintain an incontinence chart to document any patterns. Nocturnal incontinence may be altered by adjusting the timing and amount of fluid intake and the timing of diuretics. A commode or urinal near the bed is sometimes helpful. Nightlights and/or other signs that clearly identify the bathroom may reduce confusion. Other choices include use of absorbent pads or diapers for adults and protective plastic or rubber garments. Indwelling and condom catheters are popular methods of treatment, but they present a risk of infection. When behavioral approaches fail, pharmacological and surgical approaches may be indicated, but they have their risks.

The most common causes of bowel incontinence are neurogenic and overflow incontinence. Neurogenic incontinence, characterized by one or two formed stools per day, results from spontaneous rectal contractions. Overflow incontinence usually results from long-standing constipation and presents as frequent fecal staining or liquid to semi-formed stools.

There are few scientific studies on the control of fecal incontinence, and recommendations are empirical. The following recommendations are provided by Dr. Carol Winograd, a geriatrician at Stanford University. Patients should be given at least 2 liters of fluid per day, along with a diet rich in bulk. This may be initiated with a teaspoon of flaked bran or one Wasa high-fiber cracker per day. These are increased until a soft stool is produced. One teaspoon of psyllium hydrophilic mucilloid (Metamucil) in 16 oz. of water may also be used. Impaction may occur, however, if too little water is used. If bulk and fluids are inadequate, then wetting agents such as dioctyl sodium sulfosuccinate up to 500 mg. per day or senna derivatives may be used. Lactulose (15–30 mg.) is also sometimes helpful.

Included in the treatment of overflow fecal incontinence is a simultaneous emptying of the colon. This may be accomplished with phosphate enemas daily until there is no fecal return, a procedure that may take up to two weeks. Glycerine or bisacodyl suppositories have also been advocated. Long-term laxative use is not recommended.

Summary

In this chapter we have tried to present treatment and management strategies for some of the more common behavorial and mood changes associated with AD. Although presently these strategies are based more on clinical experience than research, we hope that patients and families may benefit from the interventions. As with many other illnesses, such as diabetes and arthritis, there is currently no cure for AD. However, this does not mean that the situation is hopeless. With the assistance of knowledgeable, empathic health-care personnel, the burden of caring for Alzheimer victims may be significantly diminished.

Glossary

anomia inability to find the right word for an object even though that object is accurately perceived.

aphasia impairment or absence of speech or written communication due to brain dysfunctions.

cognition that operation of the mind by which we become aware of objects of thought or perception, including understanding and reasoning.

delusion a false personal belief that is firmly sustained despite all evidence to the contrary.

hallucination a strongly experienced false perception of objects or voices that are not apparent to anyone else.

incontinence inability to control urine or bowel elimination.

insomnia inability to sleep in the absence of obvious impediments such as noise or bright lights. It may vary in degree from an occasional interruption of sleep to complete wakefulness.

paranoia a suspicion of others that is not based in reality.

paraphasia a form of aphasia in which a person substitutes one word or syllable for another and jumbles his or her words and sentences, making speech unintelligible.

physiology the science that studies the functions of the living organism and its parts.

senescent growing old.

target symptoms symptoms that should be treated.

References

Alzheimer, A. (trans. L. Jarvik and H. Greenson). 1987. About a peculiar disease of the cerebral cortex. *Alzheimer Diseasse and Associated Disorders—An International Journal.* 1:7–8.

Appell, J., Kertesz, A., Fishman, M. 1982. A study of language functioning in Alzheimer's patients. *Brain Lang.* 17:73–91.

Cummings, J. L., and Benson, D. F. 1986. Dementia of the Alzheimer type: an inventory of diagnostic clinical features. *J. Am. Geriatr. Soc.* 34:12–19.

Ferris, S. H. 1981. CNS stimulant and metabolic enhancers in the treatment of senile dementia. In: Crook, T., and Gershon, S. (eds.). *Strategies for the development of an effective treatment for senile dementia.* New Canaan: Mark Powley Associates, pp. 173–88.

La Rue, A. et al. 1986. Clinical tests of memory in dementia, depression, and healthy aging. *J. Psychol. Aging* 1:69–77.

Reifler, B. V., Larson, E., and Hanley, R. 1982. Coexistence of cognitive impairment and depression in geriatric outpatients. *Am. J. Psychiatry* 139:623–26.

Schwartz, M. F., Marin, O. S., and Saffran, E. M. 1979. Dissociations of language function in dementia: a case study. *Brain Lang.* 7:277–306.

Winograd, C. H., and Jarvik, L. F. 1986. Physician management of the demented patient. *J. Am. Geriatr. Soc.* 34:295–308.

CHAPTER TEN

Emergency Situations for Patients and Caregivers

Elaine S. Yatzkan, A.C.S.W.

LIVING WITH AND CARING FOR a victim of Alzheimer's disease (AD) can make many days seem like emergencies. But it is necessary to differentiate between a feeling of crisis—believing that you just cannot go on anymore—and an actual emergency. Even when it feels as if you cannot continue caregiving for another day because you are simply worn out and at the end of your rope, you will probably get through the day just as you have during the preceding months or years. However, when you feel this extreme anxiety, you are at a point when it is time to take action to prevent a real emergency from occurring. Taking action may mean calling a meeting with other family members to discuss plans for the immediate and long-range future; arranging a consultation with a physician to prescribe medication to alleviate the patient's problem; arranging for some time away from the patient (respite); or considering placement of the patient in a residential-care setting. An emergency is a crisis that requires *immediate* intervention. In the course of

146

providing care for a person with dementia, different kinds of emergencies may arise from time to time.

What to Do If the Patient Gets Lost

There are a number of emergencies that can happen to the Alzheimer patient just because his or her judgment is impaired. One of the most common emergencies—fortunately one that often gets resolved quickly—occurs when the dementia patient gets lost. A patient can disappear in a split second when the caregiver's attention is even momentarily distracted. Once lost, many dementia patients do not have the mental capacity to either telephone for help or seek assistance from the police. Along the way, the patient may have lost his or her wallet or purse with identifying information. Frequently he or she will not remember his or her address or phone number, particularly under stress. An identification bracelet is of great help in this kind of situation.

If the patient is lost, it is necessary for caregivers to mobilize help quickly to search for the patient. Caregivers should carry with them a recent picture of the dementia victim so that police and others involved in the search know for whom they are looking. It is also helpful to have more than one recent photo available at home. If the police and any others are initially unwilling to help in the search, the caregiver needs to make them aware of how serious it is for a dementia patient to be lost. Caregivers have sometimes been told that the Missing Persons Bureau will not become involved until the person has been gone for twenty-four hours. You must not accept this. You may need to quickly educate local police or others who may be involved as to the nature of dementing illness. Most people assume that normal-looking adults know what they are doing and understand the consequences of their acts. Caregivers know that the dementia patient they are caring for is not able to protect himself or herself adequately. Community help must therefore be mobilized to search for the missing patient immediately. It is important to keep a telephone line free so that when the patient is found you can be notified. Most lost patients are found and returned within a relatively brief period of time. Once a patient has been gone for more than a day, publicity becomes very important. Getting a local TV station to show the person's picture on the air or having the newspaper print the photo can be extremely helpful. Putting up signs with a reproduction of the patient's picture may help to mobilize the community. Hospitals, nursing homes, mental-health facilities, or other places where someone might bring a lost, confused adult should be alerted. Churches and synagogues should be contacted, as well, as congregants may be potential members of search parties, if asked.

What to Do If the Patient Ingests a Poisonous Substance

Another emergency caused by the patient's cognitive impairment occurs when the patient mistakenly ingests a potentially toxic product such as poison, medication, paint, bleach, or any other nonedible substance. A poison-control center exists in most cities; call 911 or the operator for assistance if you need help in reaching the local chapter or the national center. Both phone numbers should be posted near the telephone. Call the patient's doctor immediately. The patient will need immediate help and may have to be rushed to the hospital. A good preventive measure is to keep poisonous substances—furniture polish, paint thinner, drain opener—in a locked cabinet to which the patient has no access.

Patient Injury

If the Alzheimer patient has a bad fall, is struck by a heavy object, or cuts himself or herself deeply, it should be treated as an emergency. Remember that dementia patients cannot always articulate pain adequately and may be unable to tell the caregiver if something is wrong. Also, many demented patients have lost the ability to interpret their body's cues and may no longer understand that something is painful or that they don't feel well. Therefore, the caregiver must be extra cautious and should contact a doctor even if the patient doesn't complain. When in doubt, err on the side of caution.

Patient Illness

Dementia patients can and do have other illnesses besides dementia, and they can get acutely ill. They can have a high fever, an emergency appendicitis, a gall-bladder attack, kidney stones, a heart attack, a stroke—all of the various emergencies that can happen to anyone. It can be difficult for the caregiver to recognize the severity of the condition if the patient cannot adequately verbalize the problem. If the patient seems to be in acute pain, has difficulty breathing, is falling, or suddenly spikes a high temperature, the problem must be treated as an emergency, and a doctor should be called immediately. The patient's condition may necessitate calling an ambulance in order to get to a hospital quickly.

Victimization of the Patient

Because dementia patients do not always understand their environment, they can easily be victimized by unscrupulous people. This is particularly true of those patients who are still living alone or who are left unsupervised. The patient could be persuaded to turn over bankbooks, sign documents he or she does not understand, give away money, or pay more than once for the same item. A confused patient could easily be given the wrong change or misplace large sums of money, jewelry, or other possessions. A demented patient could allow a stranger into his or her home and be robbed or otherwise abused. If family, friends, or neighbors observe that a demented person is being victimized in any of these or other ways, it must be considered an emergency. You should involve close family immediately and contact the police. Legal interventions can be implemented to protect a demented person; these include conservatorships, legal guardianship, and involvement of the Protective Services Agency (see chapter 18).

What to Do If the Patient Gets Arrested

A dementia patient may unwittingly perform an illegal act and get arrested. Some of the common situations include being arrested for shoplifting, because he or she no longer understands that payment is required; urinating or disrobing in a public place; or becoming agitated and aggressive due to confusion. The police and the complainants may need to be educated regarding dementia; in some cases, legal counsel may be required to resolve the problem. Under no circumstances can the demented person be counted on to handle the situation alone, for he or she probably does not understand the incident or may even forget that it ever happened. Patients cannot properly defend themselves, and they need to be "rescued" immediately. Once the initial emergency is handled, it is necessary to assess how the problem happened and take action to prevent any recurrences. The person may need more supervision or medication to diminish agitation.

Violence/Abuse

Occasionally an Alzheimer patient may have an episode of violence and severe unmanageability. This may occur in response to a situation that is overly stimulating and confusing, but it can also be totally unprovoked, the result of brain damage from the dementing illness. Being struck by a person to whom one devotes so much attention can be emotionally devastating for caregivers. It is important to gain enough perspective to realize that the patient is unable to comprehend his or her actions realistically and probably will not remember having been violent. But the caregiver, or other persons, could potentially be seriously injured, so violence must be treated as an emergency and immediately contained. It may be necessary to call the police for assistance if the situation appears dangerous. Police may help to bring the patient to a hospital emergency room where the patient can be sedated, or the patient's doctor may prescribe medication to calm the patient.

Conversely, a caregiver may become so overwrought by the stress of caregiving that he or she may become violent toward the patient. If the patient is injured, it is essential to get help immediately, either at a hospital emergency room or from a family doctor. After the initial emergency it is imperative that the caregiver get some form of psychological help. A caregiver who has lost control of his or her emotions and injured a patient has overreached the limits of his or her caregiving ability and may need to consider placing the patient for temporary respite or long-term care. Clearly, help for the caregiver is in order.

Caregiver Illness

One of the emergencies that caregivers tend to fear most is their own acute illness or death, which would leave the patient suddenly uncared for. This is a very real concern even for younger caregivers. Thus, before a crisis arises, it would be wise to prepare for just such an emergency.

It is very important that you share information about your situation with a family member, a trusted friend, or perhaps a close neighbor. By just being aware of any potential problems, they may be able to assist you. Keeping the illness a secret (beyond the very early, perhaps uncertain, times) will deprive both patient and family of the social support that is needed.

One important preparatory step is to have emergency phone numbers posted next to your telephone. These numbers should include those of a relative or friend to call in case of emergency, your doctor, and any others you feel would be important in such an emergency. Some families prepare what is called a "vial of life," a special list of important phone numbers and instructions in case of emergency, which is placed in a small plastic vial and taped on an inside wall of the refrigerator where the patient won't see and remove it. (This is an accepted practice and many emergency units will know to check for the vial). The vial instructions should state that the person for whom you are caring has a dementing illness and cannot be left alone in the event you need to be hospitalized. You should also list names and phone numbers of people who could take over care of the patient. It is essential that you note in a prominent place that a vial of life can be found in the refrigerator or other place for safekeeping. Otherwise, few untrained people may think to look there for it. Table 10.1 provides a list of suggested phone numbers to be completed and kept by your telephone.

If you, as a caregiver, must go to the hospital and no neighbor, friend, or family member can be found to take over immediately, it is usually preferable to have the dementia patient go along in the ambulance with you rather than be left home alone. Most hospitals have a Social Service Department or some person who can make temporary arrangements for the demented person while the caregiver is acutely ill. Possible arrangements may include finding an

Table 10.1

Emergency Resource List

A. *Emergency Numbers*

   Police _____

   Paramedic/rescue squad _____

   Hospital emergency room _____

   Mental-health center/clinic _____

   Crisis-intervention services _____

   Suicide hotline _____

   Protective services _____

   Poison control center(s) _____

   Fire department _____

   Local bar association (for lawyer referral) _____

   Ombudsman _____

B. *Respite Services*

   In-home aides/attendants _____

   Temporary respite facility _____

   Nursing homes that will accept short-term patients _____

   _____

C. *Other Important Numbers*

   Primary physician _____

   Relatives _____

   Friends _____

   Neighbors _____

   Alzheimer's Disease and Related
   Disorders Association (ADRDA) ___1-800-621-0379 (In Illinois: 1-800-572-6037)___ for toll-free information

   Local ADRDA chapter _____

   Autopsy Network representative—chapter _____

                              regional _____

available family member, temporary hospitalization, temporary nursing-home placement, or other respite.

The importance of an identification bracelet cannot be overemphasized. The ID bracelet is invaluable for the patient and can also be helpful in a caregiver emergency. If the caregiver were to become acutely ill on the street, for example, no one might notice anything unusual about the Alzheimer patient accompanying him or her, because Alzheimer patients frequently appear normal and have good social skills. An ID bracelet that alerts onlookers or emergency personnel to the Alzheimer patient's illness might make the difference between the patient's being cared for or his or her being left to fend for himself or herself. ID bracelets are available to order at most drugstores and pharmacies or can be purchased at a jewelry store, which will engrave it with the appropriate information.

Suicidal Feelings

Caregiving can be extremely stressful. Caregivers must often deal with their own feelings of anger, frustration, and depression and may seek professional help in dealing with their emotional pain. In rare instances, a caregiver may develop suicidal feelings. This is indeed an emergency situation, and help needs to be summoned immediately. Family and/or friends need to make themselves available to take over the care of the dementia patient and to get help for the distraught caregiver. A family doctor may be called in a suicidal emergency. If the caregiver is receiving psychiatric care, the therapist should be contacted. Police emergency personnel can be called and will usually respond promptly. In larger communities many hospitals have psychiatric emergency rooms. If not, a regular hospital emergency room can handle this emotional crisis.

What to Do If the Nursing Home Threatens to Discharge the Patient

Another emergency situation that may occur for a caregiver is if the nursing home in which the patient resides attempts to discharge the patient back to the caregiver. If the nursing-home staff finds the patient difficult to manage, it is highly likely that the at-home caregiver will find the patient impossible to manage, as well. Such a discharge should be vigorously resisted. The patient's doctor should be contacted. It also may be necessary for the family that is being pressured to seek immediate legal counsel or contact the nursing-home ombudsman in the community, if one is available. The family and the nursing home may need to confer on establishing a management plan within the nursing home that reduces the patient's difficulty and makes his or her behavior acceptable. Prescribing an appropriate medication may make the patient more manageable in the nursing home. For some patients a vigorous exercise regime, with long walks, the space to pace back and forth, or other environmental manipulations, may bring about a dramatic improvement in behavior.

The United States Federal Code on Standard Patient Rights for patients in skilled nursing facilities (43 CFR Section 405 1121K) deals with the issue of involuntary nursing-home discharge. It states that a resident of a skilled nursing facility may be transferred or discharged only for medical reasons, for his or her welfare or that of other patients, or for nonpayment of his or her stay. The patient is to be given reasonable advance notice to ensure an orderly transfer or discharge. When (as is the case with Alzheimer patients) a resident is incompetent and medically incapable of understanding his or her rights, or where communication barriers exist (as is frequently the case with AD patients), the right of transfer and discharge evolves to the next of kin or the sponsoring agency. Each state has its own patient-care investigatory and regulating units, and thus procedures differ somewhat from one state to another. The Department of Health in your state can provide help and guidance should the issue of involuntary discharge occur.

Other Urgent Situations

There are a number of other situations that are not emergencies but are urgent matters requiring prompt attention. If the patient stops eating or drinking or has repeated falls, medical treatment is essential. The patient's doctor should be contacted, or another source of medical care must be sought. Such a situation can soon change from an urgent one to a full-fledged emergency if not handled immediately. Drug reactions, either from new medications or from high levels of previously prescribed medications, require immediate attention. If a drug reaction is suspected, call your physician immediately and report what you observe. Caregivers should be familiar with signs of adverse reactions to medications, including unusual drowsiness or agitation; sudden changes in balance or walking; unexplained falling; rash or itching; or gastrointestinal upset. The prescribing physician and your pharmacist can supply you with this information.

Other urgent situations occur when the caregiver feels at his or her wit's end. Some caregivers make every attempt, usually unsuccessfully, to leave the patient in a hospital emergency room in order to get some respite or to find additional help. When a caregiver feels this distraught, he or she must seek guidance. There are usually a number of options available. Most Alzheimer's Disease and Related Disorders Association (ADRDA) chapters have support groups where people can share their problems and get assistance (see chapter 13). The family doctor may be a source of comfort, or a therapist conducting individual or group counsel-

Table 10.2

**Emergency Situations
for Alzheimer Patients and Their Caregivers**

I. Emergencies That May Happen to the Patient

PROBLEM	DISPOSITION	PREVENTIVE MEASURES
a. Patient gets sick—fever, convulsions, heart attack, stroke—or becomes injured.	Medical—family doctor, rescue squad, hospital emergency room.	a. Have emergency numbers available. • Have knowledge of first-aid measures. • Make sure patient has regular medical care. • Check environment for potential hazards.
b. Patient gets violent or uncontrollably agitated.	Medical—family doctor, hospital emergency room; may require police assistance.	b. Have emergency numbers available. • Consult physician for medication and have it available. • Keep environment calm.
c. Patient ingests poison or foreign object.	Medical—family doctor, poison control center, hospital emergency room.	c. Have emergency numbers available. • Keep poisonous substances in a locked cabinet.

157

Table 10.2 (cont.)

**Emergency Situations
for Alzheimer Patients and Their Caregivers**

I. Emergencies That May Happen to the Patient

PROBLEM	DISPOSITION	PREVENTIVE MEASURES
d. Patient abused by caregiver—patient gets hurt.	Medical—family doctor, hospital emergency room, counseling for caregiver.	d. Have emergency numbers available. • Seek counseling *before* this happens—professional and/or support groups.
e. Patient gets lost.	Social—family, friends, neighbors, social supports, police; chapter, radio, TV, newspaper.	e. Have emergency numbers available. • Patient ID bracelet. • Locks/alarms on doors. • Don't leave patient alone.
f. Patient is victimized.	Social/legal—family, police, and legal intervention may be needed; conservatorship, guardianship; may need to involve protective services.	f. Have emergency numbers available. • Consult an attorney regarding protecting patient's interests. • Don't leave patient unsupervised. • Don't allow patient to carry large sums of money, checks, credit cards, etc.

g. Patient gets arrested/accused of crime.

Educational and legal intervention may be needed.

g. Have emergency numbers available.
   • Close supervision of patient in public places.

II. Emergencies That May Happen to the Caregiver

a. Caregiver gets sick suddenly and can't care for victim.

Family/social support—family, friends, neighbors to be contacted. Family doctor may arrange temporary hospitalization or nursing-home placement. Other respite services may be available.

a. Have important and emergency numbers available.
   • Make arrangements in advance with friends, relatives.
   • Check out temporary respite care available.

b. Caregiver is suicidal.

Medical—family doctor, hospital emergency room, mental-health-crisis team. Arrange care for patient.

b. Have important and emergency numbers available.
   • Seek professional counseling and/or support groups.

c. Caregiver dies suddenly.

Social—family, neighbor, friend, respite. Arrange care for patient.

c. Have important and emergency numbers posted by telephone.
   • Discuss emergency plans with relative, friend, etc.
   • Have all information—people to call, respite services, etc.—clearly outlined.

Table 10.2 (*cont.*)

Emergency Situations
for Alzheimer Patients and Their Caregivers

II. Emergencies That May Happen to the Caregiver

d. Nursing home tries to discharge patient for unmanageable behavior.

Social/medical—family doctor, counseling services for caregiver, ombudsman.

d. Choose the proper long-term-care facility for the patient.

• Facility should be experienced in working with Alzheimer patients.

• Keep in contact with the staff—physicians, nurses, aides.

III. Situations That Are Urgent but Not Emergencies

a. Caregiver reports that patient has stopped eating and drinking.

Medical—family doctor or other source of medical care.

a. Have important and emergency numbers available.

b. Caregiver reports that patient has been having repeated falls.

Medical—family doctor or other source of medical care.

b. Have important and emergency numbers available.

c. Caregiver reports adverse drug reaction in patient.

Medical—family doctor or other source of medical care.

c. Have important and emergency numbers available.

• Know about possible side effects of medications.

160

d. Caregiver is at wit's end.	Social/medical—family doctor, chapter, one-on-one support group, respite.	d. Seek professional counseling and/or support groups. • Use respite services to give caregiver personal time.
e. Caregiver unsuccessful in leaving patient at hospital emergency room.	Social—planning and counseling with assistance of family doctor, counseling services. Temporary placement may help.	e. Use respite services regularly. • Seek professional counseling and/or support groups.
f. Caregiver requires elective surgery or elective hospital admission.	Social—planning, temporary placement, or in-home respite to care for patient.	f. Make arrangements in advance for temporary placement.
g. Patient dies, and caregiver wants autopsy.	Medical—family doctor; refer to chapter representative and ADRDA Autopsy Network.	g. Advance planning—discuss with family members and contact ADRDA for more information.

161

ing can be very helpful. Temporary or long-term respite placement may provide a solution or at least a short-term reduction of stress. When caregivers feel at their wit's end, they need to reach out for help. Dementing illness is a very long-term problem, and even the strongest, most stoic caregiver may experience severe psychological distress.

Another urgent situation, but not an emergency, occurs when the caregiver requires elective surgery or elective hospital admission. Plans must be made for the dementia patient, who cannot stay alone. There are a number of possible options, including hiring someone to stay at home with the patient, temporary nursing-home placement, or other respite placement with a family member or good friend. It is essential that the caregiver attend to his or her own health needs and not unduly delay necessary medical treatment.

In summary, caring for a dementia patient is an ongoing stressful situation. At times, emergencies will arise that must be dealt with quickly and effectively. Often, advance planning can be done to lessen the urgency of certain situations. Use the list and summaries in this chapter as a quick reference for emergencies and urgent situations that may occur. This includes steps to follow to both prevent and solve these problems (table 10.2). The caregiver should be familiar with these and other potential problems that he or she may encounter in providing care for the Alzheimer patient. Advance planning can prevent panic and uncertainty when one is faced with unusual and stressful situations.

CHAPTER ELEVEN

Dealing with the Emotional Turmoil of Alzheimer's Disease

Renee Pollack, M.S.W.

WHEN A SERIOUS ILLNESS strikes, there is general upheaval in a family. When the diagnosis is Alzheimer's disease (AD), the emotional and physical turmoil is felt by everyone— spouses, siblings, adult children, relatives, and friends. Indeed, *no family member goes unscathed* when this slow, deteriorating illness afflicts a loved one. The physical demands of coping with a chronic illness are often overwhelming, and the psychological burdens placed on the family can be excruciatingly heavy.

If one has to summarize in a few words the effect on the family, I contend that this disease causes a "medical separation." As the disease progresses, needs diverge. The disease changes the former relationship that family members had with the patient. The AD patient needs guidance, supervision, and increasing personal care. The mate becomes more like a parent; the AD patient more like the dependent child. For the children of AD patients, roles also change, and they must assume a more parental stance with their afflicted parent. These divergent needs and changed roles create increasing distance—or may require physical separation for medical reasons. The medical separation triggers withdrawal and reluctance in the patient and a wide range of feelings in family caregivers. Indeed, there is usually a tremendous sense of despair for both patient and family as the patient's ability to cope with day-to-day skills begins to diminish. For the family caregiver, there is a pessimism, a sense of futility, and an exhaustion that are almost indescribable. Whether it is the sharing of day-to-day happenings or of special times, plans and dreams must be put aside. Events such as a birthday, an anniversary, a family gathering, or a friend's party take on a different meaning. These activities may bring about a sense of engulfing aloneness, with a feeling of no light after the darkness. Furthermore, the concerns and energies of relatives and friends too often become centered on the patient rather than the caring family member. People unthinkingly make inquiries regarding the progress of the patient's illness and overlook the weariness of the caregiver, who must settle down to years of living and coping with this chronic illness while figuring out ways of self-protection in the process.

The caregiver, in reevaluating his or her own life, must look at the shifting of roles caused by this deteriorating illness. Thus new responsibility suddenly takes on the highest priority and can become the overwhelming focus in each family member's life. Let's look at some of the possible role changes that may occur in the family structure.

Role Changes Within the Family

If the Alzheimer patient was the breadwinner, the family must first deal with the financial burdens caused by the illness and the patient's inability to work. Bills must be paid and insurance policies and medical coverage reviewed. In the situation of a married couple where the male spouse is the patient, a previously unemployed wife will need to evaluate her own job skills and her ability to meet her family's financial needs. Education costs for the children will need to be considered, and mortgages, rents, and outstanding debts will need to be reviewed. The role reversal takes on greater significance because of the timing of the illness and the fact that many of the medical and homemaking costs are not reimbursable. Thus, the impact in taking on the other roles becomes more stressful.

If it is the working man or woman who must take care of an afflicted spouse, he or she will have to deal with the additional emotional demands of planning for supervision and housekeeping when the spouse is home alone. In addition, he or she will have to juggle a demanding work schedule with the day-to-day issues of running the household, such as shopping, cooking, and laundry.

If the caregiver is an adult child, there is a reversal of roles between the parent and the child, with the parent now dependent on the adult child for daily physical and protective care. It can be difficult for grown children, who often live in a different geographic area with their own spouse and children, to find themselves suddenly responsible for a parent who needs day-to-day monitoring and supervision regarding even the simplest of tasks.

Individual Concerns

Spousal caregivers may be asking, What do I tell my friends? Could I have prevented this illness? Am I doing enough? What happens if I become ill, too? Who will take on the burden of caring for the Alzheimer patient? At what point do I acknowledge that I cannot do it alone? How do I get outside help? When should I place my spouse in a nursing home? How do I handle the guilt I'm feeling in this situation? How do I cope with my own life and my own needs?

Adult children, understandably, may fear the unknown of AD. Is it contagious? Is it hereditary? Is it environmental? Will it happen to me? How can I, a child, step in and take things away from my parents? How will I juggle this additional responsibility with my job, my spouse, and my children?

Adolescent and younger children may ask, Is it catching? Did I cause it? What do I tell my friends? How can I keep myself from being embarrassed? What if something happens to my well parent? What if we cannot live here anymore?

Dealing with the Illness

The impact of AD can be conceptualized by five stages of emotional reactions that family members dealing with chronically ill patients often go through. These stages may have blurred boundaries. One stage may be longer that another; some may be skipped by particular individuals; some may be experienced in varying order; some may be more painful than others.

STAGE 1: FRUSTRATION

In the earliest stage of confronting AD, often beginning before diagnosis, well family members feel a sense of disbelief, puzzlement, and discomfort. Sometimes it seems clear that something inexplicable is happening to the afflicted family member. At times the person seems like his or her old familiar self. Denial alternates with fear. The family feels a sense of frustration, loneliness, guilt, anger, and embarrassment in dealing with the patient. No matter what peculiarities the patient exhibits, whether it is a constant preoccupation with physical symptoms (which are often the only way patients can describe the changes that they perceive are happening to them), wandering, or inappropriate actions, the patient's dependency needs increase with time. Simultaneously, the caregiver may find himself or herself more independent and needing more space. Resentments build. The caregiver's negative feelings, usually not verbally expressed but very much on the surface, become directed toward the patient, who is unable to respond to the situation other than to continue to need help.

STAGE 2: ISOLATION

As the chronic illness develops and the physical and behavioral signs of the patient become more pronounced, the caregiver senses his or her isolation even more intensely. Friends and relatives may socialize less frequently. Telephone calls and visits may become few and far between, and the physical and emotional burdens of caring for the patient increase. As the caregiver's social outlets diminish and the responsibilities rise, exhaustion begins to mount.

STAGE 3: RESENTMENT

There comes a time when the chronically ill patient becomes partially or totally dependent on the caregiver for all the activities of daily living, such as dressing, bathing, eating, toileting, and walking. The caregiver's loneliness, exhaustion, guilt, anger, and sadness manifest themselves in a resentment that this illness is continuing with no end in sight. "Why me?" asks the caregiver, who is feeling the burden even more strongly than other family members.

STAGE 4: LETTING GO

As the patient's chronic illness continues and his or her dependency heightens, the caregiver must raise the question as to whether the patient needs to be in a different environment, such as a nursing home. The issue of giving up the role of full-time caregiver to someone else has a tremendous impact, and the caregiver often experiences an incredible sense of sadness and guilt related to abandonment. Even if the decision is less radical than institutionalization, for example, bringing housekeeping, homemaking, and nursing services into the home, the caregiver is surrendering the active role he or she has performed so steadily to someone else.

STAGE 5: RELIEF VERSUS DESPAIR

In the fifth stage of the chronic illness, the guilt, the anger, the sadness for the loss, and the relief that sometimes comes from the end of caregiving again come to the surface, and these feelings must be confronted. How? Working these feelings through by oneself is difficult; turning to a professional in resolving some of these feelings and issues allows the caregiver to talk to someone with objectivity and in a "safe" environment. It is important that these feelings be given the appropriate time and that the tears, the sadness, and the remembrances be allowed to surface as part of this mourning period.

Seeking Emotional Help

Caring for an Alzheimer patient brings many feelings to the surface—depression, guilt, anger, sadness, exhaustion, and social isolation. It is important that the family member acknowledge and confront these feelings. Because of the long-term and unrelenting nature of the disease, this is not easy. The losses continue, as does the grieving.

In the process of coping with the illness, many caregivers seek emotional support from self-help groups in their communities. Some individuals will seek additional help from professional counseling, which may help to alleviate some of the emotional pain. Professional help offers the caregiver and other family members a nonjudgmental environment where they can talk to someone skilled in dealing with difficult life situations. The professional can act as a sounding board, for he or she is trained to listen, to ask questions, to raise issues, and to guide family members through crisis periods. In some cases, for example, where a family member is experiencing a severe depression, the family may also consult a physician who can prescribe appropriate medication.

The following are some questions and answers that may serve as a guide in seeking professional help:

Q. How is counseling different from self-help support groups?

A. Professional counseling is *not* a replacement for self-help family support groups and vice versa. Self-help groups offer family members an opportunity to share common happenings, experiences, and coping tactics while adding a social dimension that is most important during these difficult times. These support groups may meet weekly or monthly and are generally led by family members. You may already be participating in a group, but this does not preclude getting additional help.

Professional counseling should optimally enhance what you talk about in these groups. It allows you to learn more about yourself with the aid a therapist skilled in helping you to deal with your emotional pain.

Q. What does it mean to say, "I need to talk to someone"? Will it mean that I can't handle my own problems, that I'm weak and unable to make decisions?

A. Quite the contrary. Saying, "I need the extra support, I need direction" is a strength. Gaining a better understanding of one's self by facing the conflicting feelings involved in caring for an Alzheimer patient could make the burden of the responsibility somewhat easier. It is *your* feelings, *your* pain, *your* sadness, *your* exhaustion, that will be dealt with in these sessions.

Q. Will I know what to talk about? What if I say the wrong things? What if I have nothing to say?

A. The professional is skilled in helping you confront and talk about personal issues and in raising appropriate questions that will guide you in the discussion. The therapist is trained to help you examine some of the conflicts you are facing, adapt to the change in life-style that has occurred, and assess the additional changes that might be necessary.

Q. Will the therapist know about AD?

A. AD is no longer a secret. Both the professional community and the public at large have become more knowledgeable about this illness as a result of extensive coverage in the media. But you must also take responsibility and be prepared to "teach" the professional about the impact of this illness on you personally and to share any educational materials or resources you might have available. It will be most helpful to share your sense of sadness or anger, your feelings of isolation and exhaustion. It is this give-and-take, this openness that comes about in the therapeutic process, that allows for effective results.

Q. I may want to share information with the therapist that the other family members know nothing about—will it be kept a secret?

A. What is said between you and the professional counselor is confidential. This material will not be shared without your express permission. You will usually be asked for written permission before any information is released.

Q. How will my talking with someone help the Alzheimer patient?

A. The patient is depending on you for his survival. If you are to perform this caregiving role, you must also care for yourself during this painfully long illness. Understanding your own emotional needs and seeking ways to fulfill them are a form of protection that must be built into your daily life. In addition, your caregiving ability is negatively affected by verbal and nonverbal behaviors, such as angry gestures, that impact on the patient. As a caregiver, you must be sensitive to the signs of burnout and physical exhaustion. The need to "let go" and allow others to take on the daily care of the Alzheimer patient, even for an interim period of time, will undoubtedly be discussed in the counseling sessions. This relief, which is often called respite, in the form of homemaker services, day care, and resources for nursing homes, may need to be planned. Many feelings, including the guilt of "letting go" and of allowing yourself some independent activities without the AD patient, may need to be discussed and worked out.

Q. Where do I find this professional counseling help?

A. Your family doctor or your Alzheimer's Disease and Related Disorders Association (ADRDA) chapter is a good source of referral. In addition, family agencies, mental-health clinics, psychiatric clinics, and hospitals are staffed by therapists skilled in working with individuals and families facing difficult situations. These therapists are generally trained in psychiatry, social work, psychology, psychiatric nursing, and counseling. They can help people talk about and plan realistically for critical life situations. There are also professionals in private practice who may offer similar services. Each community will offer a different assortment of services. Religious organizations such as Catholic Charities, Federation of Jewish Philanthropies, and Federation of Protestant Agencies operate on a nonsectarian basis and offer professional counseling services.

Q. Can we afford these services?

A. At some agencies, fees for services may be based on a sliding scale, depending on the ability to pay. You might also wish to check if your medical insurance covers counseling services and under what circumstances. Most agencies and practitioners are geared to see families as well as individuals and may have evening and/or weekend hours to meet your own hectic schedule. Fees may range widely, so it is a good idea to investigate all options carefully before making a choice.

Q. How do I ask for help?

A. You should call the counseling agency or practitioner directly to make your own arrangements. Let them know that one of your family members is an Alzheimer patient and that you would like help in dealing with how this illness is affecting you. Skilled professionals will determine how quickly you should be seen and will review the specific services that are available. Remember, therapists are also trained to respect confidentiality and will not divulge client names or personal information without both verbal and written consent.

In summary, it is important to remember that each family and each individual within the family responds in different ways to the stresses of illness and of the caregiving role. No two families are alike in their thinking and actions. Caregivers must eventually come to grips with the sadness of the illness and the frustration in caring for the patient. Professional counseling may be an important source of help in this regard. Caregivers must be self-protective during this painfully long, deteriorating illness and seek ways to mobilize inner resources and strengths they may never have known they have.

CHAPTER TWELVE

The Forgotten Victims: Adolescents and Young Adults Dealing with Alzheimer's Disease

*Lesley Arshonsky; Harriet Adelstein, M.A.,
O.T.R.; and Kathleen Stauber, Ph.D.*

ALTHOUGH THE VAST MAJORITY of persons with Alzheimer's disease (AD) are over sixty-five, there are some 60,000 afflicted persons who are less than sixty-five. In some of these cases there are children, adolescents, or young adults in the household. In other cases, the young children or adolescents are grandchildren, who are strongly affected by the illness of a beloved grandparent, although they may not live within the same household. Whether the patient is living at home or is institutionalized, the children are faced not only with the normal stages of development but also with the abnormal situation of coping with a family member who is ill.

The young adult children, adolescents, and grandchildren of patients are often overlooked—the "forgotten victims." Since the adult family caregiver is burdened with a change

173

in roles, new financial responsibilities, and his or her own emotional ups and downs, there may be little time left to recognize the issues this disease causes for their children and grandchildren. This chapter focuses on these "forgotten victims" by describing how Alzheimer's disease can affect younger family members, the concerns children may have, and how you can best deal with them.

Some of the specific problems for adolescents and young adults that are a direct result of the disease include: role reversals, no appropriate role models, anger at the disruption in their lives, and issues of grief and loss. Following are some case histories that highlight these problems:

Jill was a fourteen-year-old who was in her freshman year in high school. The majority of her time was spent thinking about boys, popularity, grades, and clothes. She was the baby of the family, which consisted of three older sisters and parents who had been "models" in terms of their relationship to each other and to the children. Jill's dad was fifty-four and mom forty-eight when the diagnosis of AD was made in her father. Both worked well together in the family business. From the outside, everything looked fine.

Things started to fall apart for Jill when her father began to have minor car accidents fairly regularly and these incidents never seemed to bother him. His personality started changing in a variety of ways—he was becoming aware that he could not do everyday tasks, and he began to constantly question why he could not do these routine things. He would only ask questions of Jill's mother, however, and her mother covered up for her husband's failings without discussing anything about his illness with the rest of the family.

Her mother's priorities and behaviors began to change. Whereas her children used to be the focal point of her life, Jill's mother was now forced to assume more responsibilities in running the family business. She became less tolerant and understanding of the needs of her children. The situation became very confusing for Jill.

Jill noticed changes in her sisters' behaviors. One sister started withdrawing and avoided the family as much as possible. One became very depressed. The third sister took over the role of parent by taking care of her father as well as mothering Jill. Everyone's actions were changing without any explanations.

Jill's behavior eventually began to change, too. This all-A student started skipping classes, failing courses, using drugs, choosing friends who were no good for her, and acting out sexually. The family noticed Jill's changes, but no one ever connected the fact that as her dad got worse, so did her behaviors. The assumption was that Jill was a typical adolescent, and the explanation everyone used was that she was just "going through a phase."

In Jill's family everyone saw her as "the baby," and there was an unwritten rule that she was too young to know or understand the truth about her father's illness. This silence, which was the family's way of protecting her, just added to her confusion and allowed her no way to figure out why her world was changing.

Another example of how the disease interferes with "normal" teenage years is when parents are aware they need outside help but cannot emotionally justify bringing strangers in to help with the role of caregiving that they perceive to be "their duty or desire." More often the case, families cannot afford the extra expense even if they would choose to hire help. Thus there may be the either unspoken or direct expectation for the children/adolescents to help with organizing the household, do added chores, take care of siblings. As the ill parent becomes less able to care for himself or herself, the child may also be expected to help with bathing, dressing, and helping the parent to eat.

It is very easy to forget, under these circumstances, that these youngsters would normally be "kids" spending time with peers, participating in sports, studying, dating, or working part-time. Instead, they find themselves in adult caregiving roles. These added responsibilities could cause resentment, negative feelings that may result in acting out behaviors, and a host of other problems.

Steven, age seventeen, lived at home with his mother, two sisters, and a fifty-five-year-old father who had been suffering with

AD for the past five years. Since the early diagnosis, one of Steven's greatest fears was that he would eventually become stricken with AD. As with the average teenager, Steven was preoccupied with decisions about what to do with his life after graduation, his job with a rock band, and the relationships between him and his friends, especially with girls.

The family had taken care of the father for five difficult years, and nursing-home placement was now necessary. At this point, Steven had to deal with the loss of his father and, at the same time, his new role of being the "man of the family." Feeling overwhelmed, he became increasingly more depressed, and when rejected by a date for the senior prom, Steven felt things were totally hopeless, and he decided to try to take his life.

Many teenagers have situations when they feel rejected. In Steven's case, the rejection, compounded by the placement of his father into a nursing home and his underlying fears of getting the disease, triggered overwhelming feelings of loss and hopelessness. His father was not there for him at an age when he needed a strong male model the most. Fortunately, Steven's mother noticed his radical change in behavior and initiated his involvement in psychiatric treatment. Once he talked with his therapist about his thoughts of suicide, he came to realize that there were other ways of resolving his problems.

Because the risk of AD becomes greater as one grows older, the more familiar situation is that of a grandchild dealing with a grandparent with AD.

Bobby's sixty-eight-year-old grandma lived at home with Bobby's aunt. She had been ill for several years and was dependent on her family for everything. When four-year-old Bobby got sick with a cold one day, he told his mother that he "needed" his medicine or he would get sick like Grandma. During visits to his grandma at his aunt's house he was frightened by her strange behaviors and would become so agitated his mother decided to skip visits for a while. At the same time, he was disturbed by his grandma's behaviors, was having nightmares, and was being seen by a psychologist. One day he announced happily that since his nightmares were going away, Grandma should go to the same doctor so he could make her AD go away.

Bobby is now six and is beginning to understand that Grandma's illness will not go away. She is in a nursing home, and since his understanding is better, he can visit without becoming frightened. He is able to help her take a drink, walk down the hall, eat ice cream, or will just sit and hold her hand. All of these interactions make him feel proud that he is "helping" Grandma.

In Bobby's case, it took his family a year before they became tuned in to his fears and emotions. Once they recognized the possible link between his agitation, nightmares, and Grandma's illness, they were able to work through his feelings by openly talking with him about his grandmother's problems as well as by finding professional help for him.

Jill, Steven, and Bobby are examples of the "forgotten victims." Young adults can be forgotten also, and just because they are older does not mean the impact of the disease on them is any less in intensity.

At twenty-one, Lynne was first beginning to develop an adult relationship with her father, since he was more comfortable with his children as they grew older. They enjoyed a friendship for the first few years she was in college, and then he began to show changes due to AD. Lynne's young adult life was considerably changed. She felt cheated because they had finally established a father-daughter adult relationship but the disease destroyed what could have been so positive. Because her mother could not physically or emotionally deal with his changes, Lynne found herself placed in the role of "becoming her parents' parent" at a young age and was not able to concentrate on establishing her own life.

Individual counseling and involvement in a caregivers' support group helped to place things in their proper perspective. Lynne used these support systems to evaluate how to help without losing sight of her own needs.

What Are Typical Responses to This Illness?

Often parents wonder whether or not their kids are normal if the children are demonstrating typical or atypical behaviors. Then, in the midst of this difficult task, a major crisis hits the family. A close family member, a grandparent, parent, aunt, or uncle, develops AD. Because it is your loved one, you are confused, bewildered, and frightened. It is a difficult and painful time for you, and if you are the caregiver for the Alzheimer victim, you are probably physically and emotionally depleted. You may think that your children are not being affected by the disease, but in all probability they are.

As a parent, grandparent, or relative, you need to understand a little about typical development so that you can have a clear understanding of what is "normal." Given that understanding, it might be easier to identify unusual or abnormal behavior in a child who is dealing with a relative who has this disease.

> Grandma Rose used to live in her daughter's home. Five-year-old Nancy throws a tantrum every time her mother leaves the house. The tantrum is because she is afraid her mother will not return, just as her grandmother seemed to disappear when her parents placed Grandma in a nursing home.

Nancy's reaction is typical of a young child, since prior to adolescence children really only see themselves as an extension of their parents. A normal child up to three years of age has a difficult time understanding that if Mommy leaves the house she will return. Having a parent or grandparent with AD complicates this typical situation, because, as in Nancy's case, her worry that someone she loved would disappear actually happened when Grandma was placed in a nursing home.

At approximately three to seven years of age "magical thinking" occurs as the child sees himself or herself as the center of the world and the child identifies with being all-powerful. At this age, although the child is beginning to individuate from parents, parents are the absolute authority and are viewed as being knowledgeable about all things. At the same time, the child does what he is told not because he knows right from wrong but because he is fearful of being punished.

A seven-year-old boy whose special grandpa has Alzheimer's thinks that the disease came magically and that he can make the disease magically disappear. When he cannot make his grandpa better, he believes that Mommy or Daddy will *definitely* know how to make it disappear. When this does not happen, the child may feel that he did something wrong and that his grandpa is being punished for his mistake.

At approximately seven to twelve years of age the child begins to reason. This is a critical step in development, because this helps the child understand why things happen. Although his or her ability to reason is beginning to develop, the child often sees things as very concrete—usually in terms of either black or white.

An eleven-year-old girl whose grandmother has Alzheimer's will be fearful that her mother will get the disease, as well. She will be concerned about her own physical condition and, because she identifies with her grandmother, might develop "psychosomatic" complaints like headaches and stomachaches. In the girl's mind her grandmother did something wrong and is being punished.

The stage of development from twelve to eighteen years old is referred to as "adolescence." One generally associates this period of growth with difficult times. Adolescents begin to be able to see the connection between their behaviors and the consequences of what they do. Prior to this stage, often with great frustration, parents do not understand why their children are unable to see the consequences of their behavior. As children enter puberty, there is a basic confusion over the physical changes that are occurring. They will have both pride and shame in their own bodies and begin to have sexual feelings about the opposite sex. This is also a time when parental support is crucial for children, yet they rebel against the support because they have realized that their parents are not perfect. As a consequence, peer support becomes most important.

A thirteen-year-old female whose mother has Alzheimer's might feel that if she had been good this would not have happened to her mother. At a time when she really needs the support of her mother to help her understand physical and emotional changes, her mother cannot fulfill this important role because of the disease.

Between the ages of sixteen and eighteen teenagers typically exhibit the most serious "acting out" behaviors, such as breaking curfew, cutting classes, drinking, experimenting with drugs. Often these behaviors are because peer-group pressure is in conflict with parental values. Because peers are so important, the adolescent will feel embarrassment and shame about the ill parent or grandparent. Frequently the adolescent will feel guilty about all of these feelings and behaviors.

A seventeen-year-old boy is disgusted and outraged when his father, who has Alzheimer's, walks around the house wearing no pants in front of his friends. He laughs along with his friends, while inside he is embarrassed and guilty; embarrassed that the father he respected could act so childlike and guilty that he hates his father at that moment.

Questions, Emotions, and Behaviors

It is important to remember that just as adults' reactions and coping skills will vary, so do those of children, adolescents, and young adults. There are two factors that affect all of them:

1. How important is the person who has Alzheimer's to this child, adolescent, or young adult?
2. How often does this child, adolescent, or young adult interact with the person with AD?

It is safe to assume that children, no matter what their age, will have questions. For example, they might ask:

1. What's happening to my relative?
2. Why is it happening?
3. Why can't medicine make them better?
4. Did I do something to make them sick?
5. Will I get it, too?
6. Will they die?
7. Who will take care of me?
8. What can I do to make it better?
9. Will this happen to my healthy parent or, in the case of a grandparent, will this happen to Mom or Dad since Grandma or Grandpa have it?
10. Why is everyone always so sad, angry?
11. Why can't things be the way they used to be?

They may exhibit a variety of emotions such as:

1. Fear: "Maybe I could get this; maybe Dad will get it; I'm afraid of Grandpa's weird behavior."
2. Guilt: "Dad asked me the same question ten times yesterday, and I feel guilty because I yelled at him."
3. Denial: "No, Mom doesn't have anything wrong with her."
4. Jealousy: "Mom has to be with Dad so much she has no time for me anymore."
5. Frustration: "I can't understand what Grandpa is trying to tell me, and I want to help."
6. Anger: "I'm so mad at Dad, I wish he were dead!"
7. Sadness: "Grandma can't bake cookies with me anymore."
8. Tension/stress: "If Dad doesn't stop pacing, I'm going to scream!"
9. Embarrassment: "We can't take Mom to restaurants anymore because she eats like a baby."

10. Overwhelming sense of responsibility: "Since Dad is so sick, I have to get a part-time job to help make ends meet."

11. Lack of willingness to take responsibility: "We did nothing but fight before she got sick, so why should I help her now?"

12. Despair, hopelessness: "We'll never be a real family again."

13. Helplessness: "I can't do anything to make Mom better."

They may exhibit many different behavioral responses/reactions and will change behaviors as the disease progresses in their relative. It is extremely important to be able to recognize these changes and then provide appropriate solutions. For example, he or she may:

1. Withdraw: stay away from the house as much as possible; refuse to go visit a grandparent.

2. Act out: exhibit a radical change in behavior such as staying out late or doing drugs.

3. Display suicidal tendencies: talk about how he or she might as well be dead; be involved in a serious accident.

4. Pretend everything is great: put on a happy front; show no sense of loss.

5. Have psychosomatic illnesses: repeated head- or stomachaches; constantly thinking and talking about having cancer or some other deadly disease.

6. Exhibit sleep disturbances: insomnia, nightmares, or sleeping during the day.

7. Develop eating disorders: overeating or refusing to eat.

8. Show changes in academic performance: good grades start to go down.

9. Run away: take off because the home situation is too much for him or her.

10. Want the ill relative to disappear: repeatedly talk about how life would be better if the victim were gone.

The way a family deals with and responds to these questions, emotions, and behaviors will naturally affect how the child will cope with AD.

What Can You Do?

The most important tool for helping adolescents and young adults to cope is your own willingness to listen and to communicate with them. They need the opportunity to ask questions and express their feelings without fear of repercussions or rejection. A nonjudgmental atmosphere will help them to become comfortable with discussions of the painful things happening in their world. Remember, younger children may have questions, but they do not always want to hear (nor can they comprehend) everything at once. Responding to what they want to know at their level is an important beginning.

Although adolescents and young adults can usually express how they feel, do not be surprised if your child does not initiate conversation. Watch for changes in behavior, inappropriate reactions, or other clues that something is on his or her mind. Be particularly alert to changes in your child's behaviors when the patient is going through a new phase. Sometimes these behaviors will be the only indication that something is wrong. This would be a good time to try to talk openly with your child.

Some children may have problems talking to their parents because they are afraid of making them sad or being a burden and may need to talk to peers in similar situations, close relatives, or counseling professionals, as in the following case:

Marla, eleven years old, had a wonderful relationship with her "Poppa." She was the first grandchild, and because of that Poppa spoiled her rotten—always doing things for her—taking her places and making her feel like a princess. When Marla was five, she began to notice changes in Poppa. At times, he was very short with her, and he did not remember how to play many of the games that they had always played together.

In the next five years, Marla became the "adult," and Poppa became the "child." Marla soon began to help him dress, walk, and eat. She would even go to the drugstore with her mom to buy diapers for him. She never really initiated talk about what was happening, and her family did not specifically bring up the subject of his illness with her. A new book for children came out about five years into her grandfather's illness. Marla was asked to read *Grandpa Doesn't Know It's Me* and was told that a lady from a newspaper would interview her about her thoughts on the book. It was the first time she had read anything about AD. On the day that the interview was to occur, Marla became quite upset over what she had read and hysterically asked her mom to call the lady and cancel the interview.

Marla's aunt had stopped at her house that same day to see how her interview was going and was surprised to find her so upset. She sat down with Marla to try and help comfort her, and suddenly five years of pent-up emotions and questions started to pour out. Marla had always been worried about discussing the things on her mind about Poppa's illness. Marla and her aunt spent one hour discussing all her other questions and feelings. At the end of their talk, Marla wanted to know how she could help the doctors find out about her Poppa's illness. They decided to raise money by having a lemonade stand entitled "Lemon-Aid for Alzheimer's Disease." Marla raised six dollars with her lemonade stand and is now very verbal about her thoughts and feelings. She even wants to write and illustrate her own book for kids about AD.

When the family was sorting through her grandfather's things, Marla asked her grandma if she could have his art kit and supplies, as this was a special interest that she shared with him. She treasures his kit and now goes around telling everyone that even though Poppa doesn't know her anymore, she will always love him and remember all the special times they have shared together.

In Marla's case, all she needed was an opportunity to talk about her feelings. Being given the book and having her aunt spend time with her demonstrated that it was all right to have questions and feelings and, most important, that it was okay to talk about them.

Some General Guidelines

1. Let your children (no matter what age) know that you care—that you know this is tough on them, as well. Sometimes we get so caught up in the disease that we forget that it is affecting our children.

2. Give them permission to say what they really feel; don't be afraid of their feelings. Sometimes it is hard to hear what a child has to say simply because they come close to saying just what is on your own mind! Unless they have a feeling that they can talk freely, however, they will hesitate to say anything at all.

3. Help your children confront and deal with their worst fears. Sometimes these are realistic fears, sometimes unrealistic, but they are certainly *very real* to the child.

4. Even though it is difficult, try to maintain as much family structure as possible. Continue to do some of the things you used to do as a family. Children gain a sense of security and self-confidence from consistent structure.

5. Try to spend some time with your child each day. It is important that he or she continue to have separate time when they are the focus of your attention. Do something your child enjoys doing with you.

6. Make family plans and carry them out. Adolescents typically balk at being asked to do anything, so don't accept "no" for an answer too readily.

7. Encourage young adults to go on with their own lives. They need support in focusing on such things as mak-

ing college plans, finding satisfactory jobs, moving into their own apartments, getting married, etc.

8. Deal with problems and conflicts—do not brush them under the rug.

9. Set aside specific times when the family can discuss responsibilities and problems. Even if your young adults are not living in the household, they will want to help, because it gives them a sense of sharing and pride. Be cautious, however, not to make "helping" the overriding concern of their lives.

As with adults, it is important for youngsters to know they are not alone and that there are others who are experiencing similar feelings. It would be a good idea to check with your local Alzheimer's Disease and Related Disorders Association (ADRDA) chapter to inquire whether it has support groups for children and adolescents and encourage your youngsters to participate if such groups are available. The focus is on providing a safe, nonjudgmental atmosphere in which kids can get together. These groups can use a variety of techniques to make it comfortable to learn about Alzheimer's and the associated problems, feelings, and situations. While some children will thrive in a group situation, others will need individual environments where they feel safe in sharing their feelings. Resources for professional help may include local family counseling agencies, schools, individual social workers or gerontologists, hospitals and other social-service providers, churches, and/or synagogues.

Especially with school-age children, it is also extremely important that you notify the child's school counselor, church or specialized activity groups, doctor, dentist, etc., that there is a serious chronic disease affecting a loved one. Unless these important service providers have information from home as to the family situation, they may not be able to lend support and counsel when needed. Conversely, it is wise to have a method for obtaining information back from these sources so you can be warned of problems that are beginning to erupt on the social or school scene. Make books, tapes, and videos available to them—they are excellent sources of information.

In summary, there are no magical solutions to help children deal with this hideous disease. There are some key elements involved, the most basic of which are honest communication and love and understanding. It is important to let children know that they are loved and that their feelings and emotions count, no matter what their age. They need to be reassured and given age-appropriate explanations of what is happening to their loved one and the family as a unit. They must have a constructive outlet for their stress and a warm, honest, and nonjudgmental environment where they may feel comfortable to express themselves. And we must always remember as adults not to let these children become the "forgotten victims."

References

Young, A. E. 1986. *What's wrong with Daddy?* Worthington, Ohio: Willowisp Press.

Frank, J. 1985. *Alzheimer's disease: the silent epidemic.* Minneapolis, Minn.: Lerner Publishing Co.

Guthrie, D. 1986. *Grandpa doesn't know it's me.* New York: Human Sciences Press, Inc. (Available through ADRDA)

CHAPTER THIRTEEN

Alzheimer Support Groups: A Framework for Survival

Jean Marks, M.A.

It's very painful to come to grips with the progression of the disease, but I gained a lot more understanding, which is so important when dealing daily, continuously, with that task. As yet there are no medical solutions—but the group helps me to accept the inevitable and, at times, to make a difficult decision. I am sure anybody who has come to know the problems of Alzheimer's disease, directly or indirectly, appreciates the support system of a family group.

Mrs. G.

ALZHEIMER FAMILY SUPPORT groups originated out of families' refusal to accept the pervasive hopelessness associated with the diagnosis. Jerome Stone, chairman of the Alzheimer's Disease and Related Disorders Association (ADRDA), and dedicated families in seven areas of the country sought to pool their information and experiences and, in the time-honored American fashion, formed an organization. Learning from the self-help movement, they established a priority for the organization from the beginning: to encourage the formation of community groups—known now as support groups—to educate families about the disease, share the latest practical information on its management, and help the stricken Alzheimer patient by "supporting" the caregiver. ADRDA now has more than one thousand support groups throughout the country.

Today, Alzheimer support groups in the United States are as varied as America's communities. Depending on the resources of the particular community, the groups organize themselves in community-specific ways. They vary in structure, organization, goals, and leadership. In some communities, groups are organized around the special needs of particular family members, for example, spouses, adult children, teenage children, and/or the bereaved. A family living in a community with a variety of support groups might explore several before deciding which group will best meet its needs. In less populated areas, the caregiving community, usually under the auspices of ADRDA, tries to meet the needs of their constituents through groups that are more heterogeneous in composition. However, no matter who the members are, there are basically two types of groups—closed and open-ended.

Closed and Open-Ended Groups

Closed groups are time limited and tend to be educational in focus. For a specified period—eight or ten weeks, perhaps—a group of caregivers will have weekly meetings, usually with the help of professionals, during which they will be taught about AD and made aware of the available service resources in the community. The format will be repeated as new families are identified in the community. These groups range in size from six to twenty-five participants. A major built-in limitation of this model, given its educational goal, seems to be how much information caregivers under stress are capable of assimilating in a short period of time and where they can turn after the group ends its sessions.

Open-ended groups have no definite termination date. They exist for as long as the group meets the needs of its participants. These groups are usually limited to ten or twelve persons. New members may not necessarily be added throughout the life of the group, although questions of when and how to admit new members have to be addressed in this model.

The organizational style of a group is determined by its leadership. Many groups are organized and led by non-professionals and are known as "peer" led. These groups tend to have mutual support as their primary goal. Other groups are led by professionals and tend to have a therapeutic orientation, while still others are co-led by a professional and a lay family member. Sensitive leadership is crucial. The focus of the group may be education, mutual support, counseling, or a combination of all these services.

While some persons may immediately find a support group calming, some persons find their first support-group meeting a difficult experience. Hearing the vivid details of someone else's difficulties may be upsetting. This may be especially problematic where groups are open-ended and persons enter at different times.

To solve this difficulty, some ADRDA chapters have developed an orientation program whereby the newly interested caregiver may be invited to a special orientation meeting in preparation for being introduced to the ongoing group. At this meeting, the support-group leader outlines the classic course of the disease and hears from the family member his or her more immediate and pressing problems. Caregivers may be given reading materials regarding the disease and its management and, possibly, referrals to other resources in the community. The material covered in the orientation meeting may provide the new member with more realistic expectations. After this orientation session, some persons may decide to postpone their entry into an ongoing group, while still others may decide to seek individual counseling instead of, or in addition to, the support groups.

What Do Support Groups Do?

Support groups may serve different purposes for family members at different times during the course of the illness and thus may be used in different ways. In general, however, they serve to provide a unique forum for the family member to deal intellectually and emotionally with AD.

The normalization of dealing with AD is an important part of the group experience. Members of a group no longer feel that they are alone in their misery. This process is also known as the universality of group experience. Group participation provides a nonthreatening environment in which members can express their ambivalent and negative feelings toward both their impaired family member and the stressful caregiving role they may find themselves in.

Intertwined with the experience of universality is instilling and maintaining hope in the caregiver. By meeting with more experienced caregivers, group members learn that there is life after caregiving (and during caregiving) and are encouraged to plan for a purposeful personal future. A support group may also offer the opportunity to establish new relationships. The group as a whole and individual group members can become the basis for a new social network.

Underlying the support group movement are the following basic premises:

1. The person responsible for the patient's care does not also have to become a victim of the disease; indeed, must *not* become a victim.
2. Some strategies for coping with behaviors exhibited by the Alzheimer victim work better than others.

3. There are ways through the labyrinth of planning and finding resources to lessen the weight of the caregiving burden.

4. Caregivers must restructure their own lives.

How Do Support Groups Work?

Very simply, support groups are composed of persons who are living, or have lived through, the experience of having a family member with AD. They share the collective wisdom of what is known about the management of the disease. They lessen the burden of caregiving by returning some measure of control to the caregiver through knowledge of what to expect from the disease and knowledge of what the caregiver might expect from himself or herself. They provide a forum for rebuilding one's support network.

KNOWLEDGE

As the disease progresses and the patient regresses, caregiver and victim must constantly adjust to new realities. In the early stages of the disease and in the early stages of the family member's new role as caregiver, support groups try to keep pace with the caregiver's urgent need to know.

In subsequent meetings, with the help of the group members, the blank pages of the unknown and unpredictable disease will begin to be filled in. For the first time, many caregivers are able to steady their emotional seesaw in response to the Alzheimer relative. It is not until the caregiver really knows the illness that he or she can begin to fashion appropriate responses to the patient's behavior. During this early stage, an enormous amount of new learning takes place for the caregiver.

A NETWORK

Some of this new learning can be obtained from sources other than a support group: books and videotapes available from ADRDA chapters, conferences for caregivers, and educational meetings held regularly in many communities. However, there is no substitute for the personal involvement in support groups. In the long middle stage of the disease, the support group may serve its most vital function: that of a community of other people with shared experiences. These are people in the same boat who have learned the new language of the disease and its management, who have learned new strategies for getting through the days and nights, who have solved early problems and have adapted to their new role as caregiver. No longer thrown by each new manifestation of the disease, support-group members achieve and maintain some small emotional distance from the turmoil created by the disease and begin to restructure their own lives.

POSITIVE REINFORCEMENT

This new knowledge and new learning often leave the caregiver in an isolated place. The caregiver's knowledge has outstripped the knowledge of friends, neighbors, and other relatives. When outsiders encounter the Alzheimer patient, they see the result of hard-earned coping skills on the part of the caregiver: a well-groomed, nonagitated patient whose social facade, often still intact, functions at a minimal level in a nonthreatening controlled situation. For each social encounter, the caregiver has set the stage, dressed the actor, choreographed the occasion and played all of the parts, and is left at the end of the encounter lonely and bereft. Outsiders—friends, distant relatives, other family members—see only the successful outcome and may wonder, really, what all the fuss is about. The rewards of trying to maintain "life as before" are simply too small for the caregiver to recreate the facade with any regularity. As the disease progresses, outsiders may seldom extend invitations, and the caregiver rarely accepts them. The caregiver and the demented relative become more and more isolated. The support group becomes the only place where the caregiver receives affirmation of heroic tasks completed and a sense of positive reinforcement.

SHARED FEELINGS

It is in a support group that extraordinary events and feelings are the stuff of the ordinary for all people present. In the support group, caregiving members find that there is no feeling alien to the caregiver of a demented person. Group members know that the desire to abandon their patients fights with the need to stay and find the renewed strength to carry on. Other caregivers recognize the feeling that results from the conflict between one's instinct for self-preservation and promises made and love remembered. Participants may "hate" the position they find themselves in. Whatever the language used by the groups, there is a shared experiential understanding of the unfairness of AD. There is comfort in shared tragedy. There is victory in each successfully learned coping mechanism. There is hope in the survival of more experienced caregivers who have stayed the course. There is solace derived from sharing discomforting feelings in a safe, accepting, and confidential environment.

PRACTICAL INFORMATION

In the later stages of the disease and the caregiving tasks, other issues surface. These may include practical issues of how to turn the home into a mini-nursing home, or financial and emotional issues of whether to try to place the relative in a long-term-care facility. Accompanying these decisions are a host of subtle and powerful emotional concerns. The need for the caregiver to "let go" is pitted against the patient's increasing dependency. The bereavement process from diagnosis to death and beyond is enormously complex for the family member.

In some communities, caregiving family members have access to professionals for emotional support and guidance. There are physicians who are knowledgeable about the management of the disease and who have time to guide family members through its long course. There are also trained psychologists, nurses, social workers, and other mental-health professionals who are experienced regarding the family dynamics of AD, but in many communities the primary source of help for the caregiver comes from the other caregivers they meet week after week in their support groups.

What to Look for in a Support Group

Once you make the decision to find a support group, your local ADRDA chapter can be helpful in steering the family to groups in your area. As indicated earlier, groups are structured differently in terms of leadership style and goals.

SPONSORSHIP/LEADERSHIP

Potential group members should first explore practical issues such as the time and place of support-group meetings. In addition, family members should ask questions about the origin and leadership of the group: Under whose auspices is the group functioning? Is it connected to ADRDA, to a medical school, or to a mental-health clinic? Have the leaders (professional or lay) had any special training? Is there any supervision of the group leaders? The accessibility of community resources, or people knowledgeable about AD, may differ across groups, and therefore it is important that a group fit the family member's needs.

COMPOSITION

The potential group member should determine the composition of the group before joining. A child of an Alzheimer patient may feel out of place in a group of spouses. Although they all may be primary caregivers, issues that come up for discussion may be particular to the relationship of caregiver to patient. Similarly, it is important to determine if most group members are still caring for their patient at home or if their patient is in a nursing home. On the other hand, group heterogeneity may be effectively handled by a skilled group leader.

Some ADRDA chapters have developed specialized support groups, for example, groups for grandchildren, adolescent children, and postbereavement groups.

GOALS/TIME COMMITMENT

Potential group members should learn *beforehand* what is expected of them. Is the group time-limited or open-ended? Is it educational only, or is it a mutual support group in which members are expected to share feelings and experiences? Some people may find themselves attending support groups intermittently for varying times through the course of the illness and may need different groups at different stages.

In summary, most of the cost of decade-long care of an incapacitated dementia patient is borne by families. In this grim reality the caregiver has an excellent source for stability and emotional renewal: Alzheimer support groups. Although they can never bear all the weight of the unmet needs of the Alzheimer caregiver, support groups are, in many communities, the sole lighthouse in an otherwise bleak and barren landscape. Until the cause and cure of AD are discovered, until a broad spectrum of services is available in all communities, until there is better financing for Alzheimer services, the Alzheimer support groups provide an essential framework for survival for Alzheimer families.

For information about the Alzheimer support group nearest you, call the toll-free number of ADRDA: 1-800-621-0379; or 1-800-572-6037 in Illinois.

CHAPTER FOURTEEN

Services for Alzheimer Patients and Their Families

Rochelle Lipkowitz, R.N., M.S.

THE TOLL THAT DEMENTING illness takes on Alzheimer patients and their families can be influenced by recognizing the emotional and practical difficulties that develop as the disease progresses. Our present health-care system provides at best only a fragmented approach to meeting the needs of victims of dementing illness and their families. In many areas of our country, there is little or no aid available. In other areas, the recent interest in Alzheimer's disease (AD) has stimulated the development of services for victims and their families. This chapter will outline the full range of services that may be required. Guidelines will be offered that may prove helpful to those involved in the care of Alzheimer patients.

Caring for an Alzheimer patient at home requires knowledge, motivation, and skills that are probably new to most families. To determine their ability to provide care and the resources available, a family must first examine their current situation, both physical and emotional, their knowledge of the illness and its ramifications, and their previous experience in coping in times of hardship and stress. The following questions are provided to help families and those working with them to focus their thinking and to determine their strengths and needs. A self-assessment questionnaire is included at the end of this chapter to use as a supplement when addressing these questions.

Questions to Think About

1. *Has the patient had a complete diagnostic workup?* A complete evaluation is vital. This includes a medical and family history, physical and neurological examination, a blood test to determine any acute or reversible problems, a CT scan, an electroencephalogram (EEG), and sometimes neuropsychological testing. Denial or fear may often prevent families from seeking an adequate workup, and sometimes a reversible condition may go undetected. More information on diagnosis is available in chapter 2.

2. *What is the patient's level of function?* How bad is the memory problem? Is the patient able to care for himself? How much supervision is needed? What are the patient's hobbies? Once these questions are answered (you may need some professional help), it is possible to plan everyday activities for the patient. Many Alzheimer patients retain social functioning and well-learned skills for a long period of time. However, caregivers must have a realistic attitude about the Alzheimer patient's abilities and plan accordingly, so that he or she can experience some success with carrying out everyday activities and maintain his or her self-esteem.

3. *Do you, the family caregiver, understand the nature of the illness?* Coping with the many changes that occur in

day-to-day life is possible only if you have accurate information about the physical and mental changes caused by the illness. Adequate information is also a must for developing plans for the future. AD is an illness that is often not physically obvious for a long time. Patients may appear quite normal, and it may be hard to envision the extreme hardship ahead.

4. *Are you capable of becoming a full-time caregiver?* A person with AD requires around-the-clock companionship, then supervision, then care. Are you yourself *realistically* able to provide these services? If not, is there another family member who would be available for this? Can the responsibilities be shared among several family members, or do you need outside help?

5. *Does the patient know the diagnosis?* A frequently asked question is "What do I tell the patient?" Some families are comfortable being candid and telling the patient that AD is a neurological illness. Optimally, this is conveyed early in the course of the illness with as much hope as possible for the patient. Others are reluctant to tell the patient anything. However, informing the patient is preferable for the patient and the family: it prevents barriers from developing between the ill and well people; it gives the patient something real to hang on to rather than thinking that he or she is going crazy; and more important, it may help the patient make decisions about his or her own future. With the trend toward earlier diagnosis, more people will be informed of their illness while still able to make rational choices about who will care for them and where. This may lift the burden of decision making from any one family member.

6. *Is the patient receiving regular medical care?* As communication becomes more difficult for the patient, a knowledgeable physician who is familiar with that in-

dividual can be sensitive to detecting health problems that may develop. Other illnesses can worsen the AD and, of course, make the individual more helpless. If the patient does not have a source of regular medical care, one should be identified as soon as possible.

7. *Are there nearby relatives and friends?* Social support is essential for the caregiver. It can make the task of caring for an Alzheimer patient more endurable for a longer period of time. Not only does the caregiver require emotional support from others but also physical relief from caregiving duties. "Time away" affords the caregiver an opportunity to regain a more normal perspective on life and fortifies him or her to return to the demanding caregiver role.

8. *Are hobbies, relationships, and outside interests a source of comfort to you, the caregiver?* This question goes along with question 7. The aim for the caregiver is to begin to develop a balance in life. Caregivers must begin to look at their own relationships and outside interests and activities as their "medication." These involvements may help ward off depression and other stress-related problems. If you feel guilty about involvement in independent activities, then it is important to look at the underlying reasons for this. Alzheimer support group meetings can be helpful here, as can professional counseling.

9. *Has the family had prior experience with long-term illness?* While such exposure may have involved extreme hardship, the experience may ultimately have been strengthening. Coping styles may have emerged. Those with no experience may have considerable amounts of anxiety and depression. Prolonged anxiety and depression are harmful to both ill and well people. Talking with friends and relatives may help you to confront these feelings, and you may also want to seek

Table 14.1

Services That May Be Needed by Alzheimer Patients and Their Families

---

Services for Patients

HEALTH CARE SERVICES	SOCIALIZATION, NUTRITION	TRANSPORTATION AND ESCORT SERVICES

Inpatient
Outpatient
Emergency
Crisis teams
Research
Case management
	Senior centers
	Drop-in centers
	Friendly visiting/
	  buddy systems
	Stroke clubs
	Parkinson groups
	Congregate meals
	Meals On Wheels
		Senior centers
		Red Cross
		Community
		  programs
		Dial-A-Ride
		Office on Aging

RESPITE, HOME CARE, AND DAY CARE	RESIDENTIAL PROGRAMS	ENTITLEMENT PROGRAMS

Home attendants,
  housekeepers,
  homemakers
Visiting nurses
Rehabilitation
Nursing Home
  Without Walls
Day hospital
Day programs
	Adult homes
	Foster care
	Board and care
	Intermediate care
	Nursing homes
	VA long-term care
	Psychiatric hospitals
		Medicare
		Medicaid
		Social Security
		  disability
		Veterans' benefits
		Other health and
		  disability insurance

SOURCE: Adapted from chart published by Alzheimer's Disease and Related Disorders Association, copyright © 1985. All rights reserved.

---

out professional help. When these usually reversible conditions are treated, there can be improvement in the quality of life for all concerned.

10. *What has been the experience with previous separations or difficulties?* AD can be considered as a disease of separation. The ill person begins to withdraw as memory worsens. The well person needs more socialization and

Table 14.1 (*cont.*)

Services for Families/Caregivers

HEALTH AND MENTAL-HEALTH SERVICES	SOCIALIZATION, NUTRITION	INFORMATION, REFERRAL, AND ADVISEMENT
Refer to *services for patients* Family/mental-health agencies Private practitioners Crisis teams ADRDA support groups	Senior centers Drop-in centers Friendly visiting/ buddy systems Stroke clubs Parkinson groups Congregate meals Meals On Wheels	Office on Aging Help line/hot lines Self-help clearinghouses Practitioners/ advisers Legal services Clergy Patient advocate/ ombudsman

ADRDA	RESPITE SERVICES	ENTITLEMENT AND GOVERNMENT PROGRAMS
Local chapter Support groups Self-help groups Telephone help line Autopsy Network National office 1-800-621-0379	Day programs Respite care Hospice Temporary placement Senior vacations/ camps Friendly visitors Home care	Medicare Medicaid Social Security disability Veterans' benefits Other health and disability insurance Protective services/ State Department of Social Services

---

emotional support during this process. This separation becomes more exaggerated as the disease progresses and the needs of patient and caregiver become more divergent. A caregiver will react to this separation usually in much the same way as when he or she was confronted with other losses. Participation in self-help groups and sometimes individual counseling as well may help to ease the pain involved in this separation.

11. *Has there been legal and financial planning?* AD is an illness with a long and expensive course. Advance planning is an important management strategy (see chapters 17, 18, and 19). Professional advice is often required. Attorneys knowledgeable in health-care law and the rights of families may be able to help plan the management of the family's estate. Attorneys or accountants may advise on how money should be spent or safeguarded so that the patient and family get the most benefit. If private services are unaffordable, families might consult a public legal-services group. The local Alzheimer's Disease and Related Disorders Association (ADRDA) chapter is a good source of referral.

Completing this self-assessment questionnaire should help you identify what type of help you'll need during the course of caring for an Alzheimer family member. The following is a list of services for the patient and family. The services discussed are included in table 14.1.

Services That May Be Needed
by Alzheimer Patients

At this writing, there are few specialized AD services available in most areas, although there may be a maze of aging and community services that may be utilized by AD patients and families. Families must attempt to locate appropriate services and must evaluate them carefully. On the one hand, where there are "specialized" services, it is wise to determine what is special about them besides the name (and possibly the price). On the other hand, more widely available services may meet the needs of AD patients or may be easily adapted to do so.

Please note that the names given to a particular service or agency vary from place to place, as does the range of services offered. Additionally, patients and families will have differing needs for services at different times in the course of the illness.

HEALTH-CARE SERVICES

Regular medical care is important for maintaining health and well-being. Outpatient care is provided by local hospitals and medical schools, clinics, private physicians, and health-maintenance organizations. In addition to ongoing medical care on an outpatient basis, these agencies may provide assessment and diagnosis regarding the dementia. Once a diagnosis has been established, direct therapy with the patient may include individual support, medication, and/or group therapy.

Inpatient care for concurrent illnesses or problems associated with the dementia is usually available at general hospitals, mental hospitals, and long-term-care facilities. Your family physician may be a good first contact. Emergency treatment is available at hospital emergency rooms, through private physicians, or by calling a local police/ambulance/rescue-squad number such as 911. Since a wide and changing range of health-care services may be required through the course of the illness, there may be a need for coordination of efforts. The role of coordinator, or case manager, may be assumed by the primary family caregiver in association with the family physician or another health-care professional.

MOBILE CRISIS TEAMS

Mobile crisis teams, sometimes called community teams, serve homebound people, often living alone, who are having difficulty managing from day to day, whether as a result of a mental illness or a dementing process. The team is usually comprised of a social worker, nurse, and physician. By seeing patients in their own homes, team members are able to assess the environment for potentially dangerous situations and determine what kind of assistance is required. In the course of trying to help clients, the agency will undoubtedly have to contact family members. Unless an adequate social support network can be devised, the homebound individual may need to enter a nursing home or some other protective environment earlier in the course of a dementing illness than those who have readily available family caregivers.

PROTECTIVE SERVICES

Usually a division of the State Department of Social Services, the Protective Services Agency can provide help to impaired elderly persons who perhaps cannot manage their money, are exploited or otherwise in danger, and are resistant to accepting services. The Protective Services Agency has the legal authority to bring court action to determine whether an individual is capable of managing his or her own property or affairs, is in need of some form of legal protection, or should be committed to an institution.

RESEARCH PROGRAMS

There are clinical research programs studying the cause, risk factors, and possible treatment of some of the symptoms of AD and related disorders. Participation in these programs may provide temporary relief of symptoms, hope for the patient and family, and a setting in which there is empathy for many of the hardships families endure.

Throughout the country there are a number of programs for the administration of experimental medications to aid Alzheimer patients and patients with other forms of memory loss. The medications are *not* a cure and cannot retard the progress of the disease; however, there have been some small advances. While most programs are for memory, others are for alteration of mood (agitation or depression) and can be very helpful in easing problems of management.

Your local ADRDA chapter may maintain a list of research projects in your area, or this information may be available from your family physician, a member of the local ADRDA Medical Advisory Board, or the national ADRDA office. Local medical schools and large hospitals may provide additional information through their departments of neurology, psychiatry, and/or geriatric medicine.

SOCIALIZATION GROUPS

Senior centers provide services for older people, generally sixty and over. These services may include a hot lunch each day and a variety of social, cultural, and educational activities. Some centers may also provide counseling, transportation, social services, and limited health services. Those centers providing an expanded range of services may be called multipurpose centers.

Senior centers are ideal for the mildly demented person, as they serve to meet social needs, to provide activities to structure the day, and often, to provide a nutritious noontime meal. It is often possible for patients early in the course of AD to maintain their normal routine with some added supervision. For example, it may be necessary to provide an escort to and from the center so that the patient may benefit from this resource.

Drop-in centers are more formal programs that usually offer a chance for some social contact. They may be especially helpful for the mildly impaired person whose social skills are usually intact.

Friendly visiting and "buddy systems" are services that are usually provided by senior centers, schools, churches, synagogues, labor unions, and the local ADRDA chapter and may serve to ease the loneliness and isolation felt by many afflicted families. "Buddy systems" are informal groups of people who provide support and assistance for each other either via telephone or by home visits. These visits may provide welcome interludes for caregivers and are usually provided free of charge.

NUTRITION PROGRAMS

Nutrition programs (sometimes called congregate-meals programs) provide meals (usually lunch) in a group setting. They may be based in churches, synagogues, schools, housing projects, senior centers, and community centers.

Meals On Wheels delivers lunches (and sometimes dinners, as well) to homebound individuals. To qualify, in most instances the individual must be without assistance for shopping or preparation of meals. The daily deliveries give the patient nutrition as well as social contact with the volunteer who delivers the meals. Meals On Wheels programs are sometimes funded by the Older Americans Act through a local voluntary agency, such as a senior citizens' center, or a hospital or may be funded through other sources by various agencies.

SPECIALIZED CLUBS/GROUPS

Stroke clubs. Strokes may impair the patient's speech or mobility. In some cases, persons with multi-infarct dementia (MID), a related disorder, may benefit from participation in these programs. A stroke club focuses on improvement of function in addition to socialization and family support.

Parkinson groups. Some Alzheimer victims develop Parkinson symptoms; some Parkinson patients have dementia. And just as there are support groups for families of Alzheimer victims, there is also a network of support groups for Parkinson families. At meetings, people learn new ways of dealing with their problems and can talk to other people who understand the difficulties they are facing. In addition, there may be meetings for the patients.

Day care is a service that provides stimulation, structure, supervision, socialization, a nutritious meal, and just plain fun for dementia victims. Program designs vary widely, as do the services offered, but day care may be appropriate through much of the course of the illness. In addition, it is a good source of respite for caregivers. Day-care programs may be freestanding or held at nursing homes, hospitals, or mental-health centers. It is best to refer patients to a specialized day program for the Alzheimer patient if one exists in the area. If, however, the only available program is for patients with physical problems, it is worthwhile to try to educate that program's staff about the special needs of dementia patients. Sometimes specific days of the week can be set aside for Alzheimer patients. The patient's functional ability, need for service, and financial resources will determine which program might be appropriate. Day care is not funded by Medicare, so patients need to pay privately or be eligible for Medicaid.

A *day hospital* may provide help in caring for the more acutely ill patient. A range of health and mental-health services may be available during the day. The patient returns home for the evening and night hours. Usually day hospital attendance is limited to a specific period, generally no more than ninety days. This may be especially useful to an Alzheimer patient during a period of extreme agitation or physical illness or to a patient after a stroke or a worsening of Parkinson symptoms. Physical rehabilitation is appropriate for victims of stroke and Parkinson's disease and can often help Alzheimer patients maintain their mobility. Day hospital services may be offered through private or voluntary agencies. In certain instances, Medicare may provide limited coverage for some patients. Others need to be eligible for Medicaid or pay privately.

HOME-CARE PROGRAMS

Home care. Families may become overwhelmed by the tremendous physical and emotional burdens of caring for a patient at home, especially when he or she requires almost total help for the basic activities of daily living—bathing, dressing, grooming, toileting, and eating. Family caregivers may need different kinds of assistance with patient care. Home care is offered through private, voluntary, religious, and governmental agencies. Depending on family finances, some assistance or cost sharing may be available.

Housekeeper/homemaker services. Housekeeping is a part-time service for patients who are physically unable to perform basic household tasks but are still able to supervise the housekeeper assigned to them. Housekeepers perform such chores as marketing, cooking, cleaning, and laundering and can be invaluable to persons with early dementia who live alone. Homemakers perform housekeeping chores and more: personal care, budget management, and nutrition. These services are available from individual workers or private or public agencies.

Home-attendant programs. Home attendants perform basic household chores such as marketing and cleaning and also assist with bathing, grooming, dressing and other personal care, budget management, and nutrition. These services are available from individual workers or private or public agencies. Home attendants perform more extensive services than housekeepers; they are not necessarily full-time.

Rehabilitation services. If prescribed by a physician, rehabilitation services, such as physical therapy and speech therapy, can be obtained from a visiting-nurse service, hospital, clinic, or private practitioner.

Visiting nurses. In some areas, visiting-nurse agencies may be responsible for the home-care services. In others, they may provide evaluation of the patient and his environment, administer medications and treatments, and fill out necessary assessment forms for private and governmental agencies, if required.

Hospice. The hospice provides services that are geared toward terminal patients who are estimated to be in the last six months of life. Hospice programs often combine home care and inpatient services. When at home, the patient may be seen by a team of physicians, nurses, and social workers. Inpatient services may include laboratory tests and X rays. Counseling and support are provided to the family. Inpatient hospice programs provide humane and necessary care without seeking to extend life artificially. There is an attitude of honesty and consideration of the patient's dignity. Many hospice programs will not accept end-stage Alzheimer patients; however, this varies from program to program, so it is worth asking about admission policies. Hospice programs may be sponsored by hospitals, nursing homes, or other social-service groups.

Nursing-home services at home. Many patients need the care provided by a nursing home but may be able to receive these services at home. For example, there is a New York State initiative called the "Nursing Home Without Walls." Similar programs undoubtedly exist elsewhere under different titles. This program provides health care at home to chronically ill or disabled older adults who might otherwise have to enter a nursing home. Each patient receives a specialized coordinated plan of care approved by a physician. This plan may include doctors' visits, nurses' visits, home-health aides' services, social work, physical therapy, speech and hearing services, respiratory services, dietary consultation, personal care, laboratory tests, medical supplies, equipment and appliances, medications, rehabilitation, and occupational therapy. In other words, these programs provide services that might otherwise be obtainable only in a nursing home. There are usually well-defined requirements, both health and financial, for participation in these programs. As for all the services discussed, your local ADRDA chapter will have more information about these resources.

RESIDENTIAL PROGRAMS

Adult homes. Adult homes may be suitable for persons with mild memory loss. These homes may be privately owned or operated by voluntary or religious organizations. They provide a safe, structured, and social environment. There is, however, only minimal supervision. Residents must be able to take care of their own personal needs and get to a common dining room for meals.

Foster care/board and care. These care programs provide a home for the patient in a smaller, more personalized setting. It may be for respite or on a permanent basis. Facilities and programs differ widely from area to area. Only some states license these facilities. In all cases, family members should ascertain that the potential caregivers are able to meet the special needs of Alzheimer patients in a safe and appropriate setting.

LONG-TERM-CARE FACILITIES

Nursing homes. There comes a time for many families when nursing homes must be given serious consideration. In many cases, placement in a nursing home is a positive step. A nursing-home staff can competently interpret the needs of Alzheimer patients and cope with such problems as frequent falling, incontinence, unusual behavior, malnutrition, and infection. Nursing homes provide different levels of care, and the choice of facility should be based on the patient's needs.

There are newspaper articles and pamphlets that describe

what to look for in the selection of a nursing home. A good place to start is your local ADRDA chapter, which may have pamphlets available and/or an active nursing-home committee. The Office on Aging or State Health Department may also have information. More information is available in chapters 15 and 16 of this book.

Many homes have long waiting lists, so early planning is necessary. People often delay taking a bed in a nursing home until the "last possible moment." If the patient has a healthy spouse, some advisers may recommend that they both enter a home together, especially if they are advanced in years, but this is only one option to consider. Others prefer to have the well spouse living in his or her own home, with easy access for visitation. Younger caregivers also need information about nursing homes. They may delay placement until they feel that the time is "ripe"—that is, when the patient cannot differentiate them from other people—and any "caring" person can provide the assistance needed.

Skilled nursing facilities (SNF) provide continuous nursing service around the clock for convalescent or chronically ill patients. Registered nurses, licensed practical nurses, and nurse's aides provide services prescribed by the patient's physician. Patients may be eligible for both Medicare and Medicaid, although Medicare will provide little or no coverage for Alzheimer patients. In some places, especially in rural areas, the county assumes responsibility for long-term care.

Intermediate-care facilities (ICFs) or health-related facilities (HRFs) provide regular medical, nursing, social, and rehabilitative services in addition to room and board for people not fully capable of independent living. Patients must be ambulatory and able to participate in their own care. Supervision is limited. Intermediate-care facilities may accept Medicaid reimbursement.

Designations of levels of care vary from state to state, and some of the distinctions may be vague. It has, in fact, been recommended that the distinctions between SNFs and ICFs be abolished.

Veterans Administration (VA) long-term care. If the patient is a war veteran, some VA hospitals have units for patients with AD and related dementing disorders. Others have their own nursing-home beds. Excellent care may be available in these facilities for qualified veterans. However, services for veterans are uneven, and ADRDA is advocating for the development of a uniform policy.

Psychiatric hospitals. There are some Alzheimer patients who may develop severe psychiatric symptoms and require psychiatric care. Psychiatric hospitals may be privately owned or run by the state or county. State hospitals were once a major source for long-term care, but very few elderly patients are involved in this system at present. There are times, however, when a protected or locked facility may become necessary for an extremely disturbed patient, and a psychiatric hospital must be considered.

ENTITLEMENT PROGRAMS—MEDICARE AND MEDICAID

Medicare is a federal insurance program administered by the Social Security Administration for people sixty-five and over, people disabled for at least two years, and people suffering from chronic kidney disease. Medicare provides partial payment for acute hospital care, doctors' visits, surgical appliances and equipment, and, in very limited situations, care in certified skilled nursing homes.

Medicaid is a medical-assistance program for certain needy and low-income people of all ages. Although there is federal funding, the responsibility is shared with the states, and each state designs its own program. Medicaid benefits thus vary from state to state. In many states, Medicaid covers payment of doctors' fees, home-health aides, transportation to health services, and both skilled and intermediate levels of nursing-home care. (See chapter 19 for more detailed information on both Medicare and Medicaid.)

Services for Families/Caregivers

ALZHEIMER'S DISEASE AND RELATED DISORDERS ASSOCIATION (ADRDA)

This national association was developed to aid people concerned with AD and related disorders. It has five goals:

- to promote and support research;
- to provide education and increased public awareness about AD and related disorders;
- to develop a nationwide network of chapters;
- to provide advocacy for victims and families; and
- to reach out to families through self-help support groups and to promote services for families and victims.

Most ADRDA chapters sponsor self-help support groups, which are regularly scheduled meetings where participants gain information and emotional support. The opportunity to meet with others who are having similar experiences and share information is invaluable for many people To contact the national ADRDA office, located in Chicago, Illinois, write or call: 70 East Lake Street, Chicago, Ill. 60601; 1–800–621–0379; or 1–800–572–6037 in Illinois. You can locate the nearest ADRDA chapter by calling the toll-free 1-800 number. Your local chapter will provide information and referrals to local self-help or support groups.

INFORMATION, REFERRAL, AND ADVISEMENT

ADRDA chapter—help line/hot lines. This network is being developed nationwide. It may be the individual's first contact with the local chapter and will provide extensive information and referrals as requested by the caregiver.

Office on Aging. This coordinating and planning agency develops and monitors programs and services for the elderly. It gives information and makes referrals on needed services such as screening for Medicaid, food stamps, and employment. It also offers help in completing applications for reduced-fare cards, the Home Energy Assistance Program, and rent-stabilized and rent-controlled apartments.

Self-help clearinghouse(s). Many states have a centralized agency that maintains information about self-help groups. This agency will provide the location of such groups.

Legal services. Some attorneys are especially knowledgeable about health-care law and the rights of families. They handle many cases involving governmental benefit programs (Medicare, Medicaid, and Supplemental Security Income). There are also several organizations that provide legal services for senior citizens who are financially needy, either at no cost or at a reduced fee. The Office on Aging in your county is a good source for this information, as is your local ADRDA chapter. (See chapters 18 and 19 for more information.)

Practitioners/advisers. Participation in self-help groups is helpful to many persons. This participation does not preclude seeking more intensive individual help, as well. Various specialists, including psychologists, social workers, and nurses, treat patients and families. Treatment seeks to help the patient and family function as well as possible and to improve their quality of life throughout the course of the illness. In order to achieve these goals, practitioners provide information as needed, identify problems that can be solved, and develop specific strategies to help the patient and family cope with these problems. (More information about this type of help is contained in chapters 11 and 13.)

Clergy. Many members of the clergy have been trained or are experienced in counseling and dealing with family crises. They may provide guidance and support in some cases.

Ombudsmen. Sometimes patients or families have problems with the working of an agency and may feel that their rights are being violated. Help is available for these problems through patient advocates, or ombudsmen. Your local ADRDA chapter maintains a list of these resources in your community.

HEALTH AND MENTAL-HEALTH SERVICES

Health services. It is just as important for the caregiver to maintain his or her own health as to assure good medical services for the Alzheimer patient. Services available are similar to those described in the section on services for the Alzheimer patient.

Mental-health agencies. Help for families in coping with the emotional burdens of AD is available at outpatient clinics of psychiatric departments in major hospitals, from various family or mental-health agencies, and from private practitioners. Health professionals, including psychiatrists, psychologists, social workers, and nurses, are educated to help families during crises.

OPTIONS FOR RESPITE

Respite-care programs are useful for Alzheimer patients who live in the community with relatives or friends who assist them in their daily living activities. When, due to vacation, illness, or an unusual family situation, family or friends are unable to provide the necessary support, the patient can enter a respite program for a brief stay until the family situation returns to normal, or help can be sent into the home in areas where this service is available.

Stays in residential respite programs are often time limited, and reservations are necessary. Nursing care may be provided as well as complete food service. There may be recreational activities and a full range of health-care services. Respite services vary widely in the type of programs provided, so it is wise to investigate thoroughly. Eligibility for a respite program may be similar to that for a skilled nursing and/or health-related facility. This is determined by a medical report from the patient's doctor. Fees are most often not covered by Medicare or Medicaid.

Temporary placement of a patient in a nursing home. This is sometimes needed when formal respite programs are not available and no one is able to care for the ill person. The same standards for admission and fee scales apply to this short-term relief as would apply to long-term placement. Some nursing homes may have a minimum-stay requirement.

Senior vacation/camp programs for the caregiver. Senior citizens may apply to this specialized camp program. It provides a stimulating and educational experience in a setting away from home. This is a very popular program, as it provides an opportunity for people to socialize in a congenial setting, which may be a college or a hotel. Family members may enjoy this as a respite from the continuously hard task of caring for their ill patient at home.

Day-care programs for patients. This service offers time away for family caregivers. They usually come to feel secure knowing that their ill family members are being cared for in a safe, structured, and stimulating environment by a warm and understanding staff.

Hospice. A hospice is a service that is geared toward terminal patients who are estimated to be in the last six months of life. As described earlier in this chapter, hospice programs often provide both home care and inpatient services. Hospice programs also offer counseling and support to family members, assisting them in dealing with their grief during the end stage of the illness and beyond.

SELF-HELP GROUPS

The multitude of self-help groups that have sprung up all over our country, primarily through ADRDA, brings home the fact that families do not have to face the illness alone. These group meetings are usually led by either an interested layperson or a combination of lay and professional persons. Participation may dispel some of the hopelessness and helplessness experienced by families. They develop a new group of friends who are having similar experiences, and they need fewer words to convey their feelings. Support groups also are a source of practical information, such as how to handle the problem of the patient's diminished driving ability or when not to leave the patient alone anymore. ADRDA has developed a network of self-help groups serving families concerned with dementing illness.

AUTOPSY

ADRDA has established a national Autopsy Network to help ensure an accurate diagnosis and to provide tissue for research on AD. Almost all of the scientific information we have about this disease has been acquired through studies of autopsy tissue. It is extremely important to obtain an autopsy whenever possible. While there are often personal or religious objections to autopsy, these may be reconsidered. An autopsy can be done quickly so that funeral plans need not be delayed. This is especially true in those cases in which permission for autopsy has been granted prior to death. This type of advance planning is increasingly common and permits the family the time to explore all of their unanswered questions about this procedure in a calm and logical manner. An ADRDA chapter or regional autopsy representative can be helpful. In cases in which local or regional representatives are unreachable, a call to the national office at 1–800–621–0379 (In Illinois, 1–800–572–6937) might be suggested.

In summary, AD has a long course that imposes medical, financial, social, and emotional burdens on patients and their families and causes them to require different services at different times. Our present health-care system provides only a fragmented approach to meeting the needs of victims of dementing disease and their families. In many areas of our country, there is little or no aid available. In other areas, the recent interest in AD has stimulated the development of many new services for victims and their families. Families should become familiar with all the options available to them.

Questions to Think About

1. Has the patient had a complete *diagnostic workup?* A workup should include:

- medical history
- mental status examination
- physical exam
- neurological exam
- psychiatric examination
- blood test
- CT scan
- EEG
- psychological testing

(The process of diagnosis is described in chapter 2.)

Action Steps

- Determine what tests have been done and what they showed.
- If there has not been a complete workup, obtain a referral to a physician (neurologist, psychiatrist, geriatrician) who is experienced in working with AD.
- If you are still uncertain, you might wish to seek a second opinion.

2. What is the patient's *level of function?*

- What is his or her degree of memory loss?
- Can he or she continue to work?
- Can he or she live alone?

- Can he or she be left alone for a significant period of time?
- How much supervision and assistance does he or she require?
- Should he or she continue to drive a car?
- Is he or she in any immediate danger?

Actions Steps

- Evaluate *objectively* what the patient can and cannot do.
- Ask a friend, relative, or professional to assist you in being objective. Sometimes it's hard to step back and see things as they really are.

3. Do you, the family caregiver, understand the *nature of the illness?*

    Check your knowledge of:
    - The course of the disease—its progression, associated symptoms.
    - Physical changes that may occur in an Alzheimer patient.
    - Mental changes that may occur.
    - Needs for planning—such as financial, legal, caregiving, medical emergencies, and long-term care.
    - Needs for service—such as home attendant, day care, family counseling.

Action Steps

- Read books and articles on the disease.
- Contact your local ADRDA chapter for additional information.
- Ask questions of the health-care professionals caring for your patient. Are the symptoms typical?
- Attend support group meetings.

4. Are you capable of becoming a *full-time caregiver?*

- Can you/will you be able to provide around-the-clock companionship, supervision, and, eventually, physical care?
- Is the patient bigger than you? If so, will you be able to bathe or lift the patient if it becomes necessary?
- If the patient has difficulty sleeping at night, how will you cope with meeting your own sleep needs?
- If problems such as wandering, agitation, or paranoia become frequent issues of concern, how will you manage the patient?

Action Steps

- Determine what you are *physically* able to do. If you need help or may need help in the future, consider your options, such as specialized equipment in the home or a companion, home attendant, or nurse's aide in the home.
- Determine what you are *emotionally* able to do. Being with one person twenty-four hours a day can be emotionally draining.
- Find time for yourself—to be alone, to visit friends, to shop, or to do whatever you enjoy.

5. Does the patient *know the diagnosis?*

- What is the physician's recommendation?
- What is the likely impact on the patient?
- If you are reluctant to tell the patient, why do you think you feel this way?

Action Steps

- If the patient is able to understand the diagnosis, it is generally recommended that he or she be told. If you are uncomfortable doing this yourself, your physician (family physician, neurologist, geriatrician) can speak with your patient.

The patient should be told in order to:
- Prevent communication barriers from developing.
- Give the patient something real to hang on to rather than thinking that he or she is going crazy.
- Help the patient make decisions about his or her own future, if possible.

6. Is the patient receiving *regular medical care?*

- Is the physician familiar with the patient?
- Is he/she knowledgeable about AD?
- Is the patient seen on a regular basis?
- Do you, the caregiver, feel comfortable asking questions and discussing your patient's care with the physician?

Action Steps

- Find one physician who will be in charge of your patient's medical care. Referrals to physicians experienced in working with Alzheimer patients can be obtained from other health-care professionals, support groups, and your local ADRDA chapter.
- Come to visits with a list of questions and concerns.

7. Are there *nearby relatives and friends* who can be helpful to you and the patient in terms of:

- Assisting with chores, errands, or caregiving tasks.
- Providing relief from caregiving.
- Providing emotional support.
- Socialization (visiting, telephone calls, shared activities).

Action Steps

- Recognize that *everyone needs help.* You can't go it alone. Help comes in many forms: a visit, a ready listener, and a shoulder to cry on.
- *Ask* for help. Friends and family may not recognize your needs. They also may feel uncomfortable themselves dealing with the illness. Talk to them and educate them about the disease and problems associated with it and make specific requests, such as: "Would you be able to go with us to the dentist's appointment on Friday so that I can take him inside while you park the car?"

8. Has there been legal and financial planning?

- Have you consulted an attorney to discuss estate planning?
- Is there a living will signed by the patient?
- Have you investigated what care will be provided by Medicare, Medicaid, and private insurance? Is the patient eligible for benefits he or she is not now receiving?
- Who will take over the caregiving role if you should die or become ill?

Action Steps

- Talk to an attorney who is experienced with trusts and estates and health-care law.
- Referrals for legal services (both public and private) can be obtained from your local ADRDA chapter.

9. Are *hobbies, relationships, and outside interests* a source of comfort to you, the caregiver?

- Do you have hobbies and social relationships you enjoy?

- Do you have time to pursue them?
- Is there someone available to relieve you of your caregiving responsibilities on a regular basis?

Action Steps

- Identify what's important for you, the caregiver. What do you enjoy or wish you had more time to do?
- Set aside a certain amount of time a day or a week for *yourself.*
- Get help to relieve yourself from caregiving, whether it is an hour or a day at a time.

10. Have you and/or your family had *prior experience with long-term illness?*

- How did you deal with it emotionally? Did you become overwhelmed? Were you left to face the problem alone?
- Did you become depressed?

Action Steps

- Think about previous experiences and how you dealt with them.
- What coping mechanisms did you develop to help you deal with feelings of anxiety, stress, depression, etc.? Did you turn to other people for help? Are you able to talk about your feelings?
- Have you thought about how you will deal with issues such as separation from your loved one and loneliness?

11. What has been your experience with *previous separations or losses?*

- Were you able to separate and continue your own life?

- If you were successful, *why?* Did you manage alone or need help from others? Did you continue to pursue your own independent life (work, hobbies, friends, etc.)?
- If you found separation difficult or impossible, what did you do to help ease the loss?

Action Steps

- Think about previous experiences with long-term illness and how you dealt with them and whom you turned to.
- Write down on paper what helped you, what you needed help with, and to whom you turned.
- Identify who might help you now—a friend, a family member, a clergyman, a professional counselor, or a therapist? An Alzheimer support group?

CHAPTER FIFTEEN

Deciding on Placement for the Alzheimer Patient: One of the Most Difficult Personal Decisions

Juliet Warshauer

"WHEN IS THE RIGHT TIME to place my Alzheimer patient in a residential health-care facility?" This question has been asked over and over again by devoted families and caregivers. There is no one answer, since so many factors can influence this decision—a decision that will probably be one of the most difficult a family must make.

When I first learned that my husband had Alzheimer's disease (AD), the neurologist said, "Your husband will not recognize you in six months, so prepare now to put him in a nursing home." I replied, "Never! He will stay at home." We were both wrong. It was eight years later that I realized that never is not forever! What had necessitated this change of heart?

For eight years I had been a constant companion and then caregiver to my husband. During the last two years, I had the help of a full-time, live-in attendant. Eventually, it was impossible for the two of us to give my husband the care he required. He could not communicate, since he had not spoken a word in years. He could not control his bodily functions. It took two people to get him out of bed into a wheelchair and then into a shower. He had to be turned in bed every two hours. He had been hospitalized and had severe bedsores on his legs. These open wounds had to be dressed twice a day by a registered nurse. At home I became incapable of giving him the care he required. Eventually, my family physician helped me to make the decision. Perhaps the most convincing reason of all was that my husband did not know where he was and it no longer mattered to him who was responsible for his care.

For me, the right time for placement became very apparent when my husband's needs for care surpassed what I could provide at home; but this was late in the course of his illness. For some people, such placement may not be necessary, especially when resources and supervision are ample or, conversely, when placement would financially destroy the remaining spouse and in-home help can be arranged. Many people ask, "What am I to do about planning for care?" Following are some suggestions, based on my personal experiences and on my work as an officer of a large Alzheimer's Disease and Related Disorders Association (ADRDA) chapter.

Who Should Care for the Patient?

As the care needs of the patient increase with the progression of the disease, you must begin to ask questions about the primary caregiver. Can this person, if a family member, cope with the emotional burden of watching a loved one slowly deteriorate physically as well as mentally? Can this person continue to devote days and nights to someone who may be unable to recognize him or her and who will almost never say, "Thank you"? Does this caregiver have the physical stamina and strength to help the patient get in and out of a chair, walk, dress, bathe, and use the toilet? What is the physical condition and functional ability of the patient? Is the patient incontinent (unable to control urine, feces, or both)? Can he care for his personal needs? How great are the demands he will make on the caregiver? The family will likely want to keep their loved one at home unless the safety of the patient and/or the caregiver is endangered. As the demands increase, it may become necessary to bring in outside help.

The financial situation must be evaluated also. Can you afford to pay for additional help? How much? And for how long? Chapter 19 will help you investigate your options. Eventually, it may be necessary to have professional care around the clock. At this point, placement in a nursing home may be the best answer, but this will occur only if the family and particularly the caregiver are psychologically ready to "let go"—to relinquish the care to trained people who are not emotionally involved.

When Is It Time for Placement?

The time before placement is a time to reflect: can I give a task over to strangers that has consumed my days and nights for so long? In reality, many patients will do better in a structured environment with caring professionals to provide physical, emotional, and social care. It may be more stimulating for the patient to share meals and activities with others instead of sitting at home staring at the television. And it may be a relief to the caregiver that someone else can take over and do the job as well or maybe even better.

Some situations may dictate placement of the patient earlier in the course of illness. Some people cannot watch their loved one suffer through too many stages of this insidious disease. For them, early placement in a residential facility must be their choice. Other families have no one available to stay at home caring for the patient and supervising his well-being, and in such cases, placement is most practical and beneficial for them. Patients who live alone may require placement when they can no longer make it on their own.

Looking for a Residential-Care Facility

When the family has decided that placement is the best solution to their problem, a residential-care facility that meets the needs of the patient as well as the family must be found. First, you must recognize what your options are. For less impaired patients, there are residential programs such as foster care, board and care, adult homes, or domiciliary-care facilities. (Different states may have different names for these types of care.) For the more severely impaired patients, nursing homes may be appropriate, but there is variation in the levels of care they offer.

Nursing homes provide essentially two levels of care, that is, skilled nursing and intermediate care, and the choice of facility should be based on the patient's needs. Skilled nursing facilities (SNF) provide continuous nursing care around the clock for convalescent or chronically ill patients. Registered nurses, licensed practical nurses, and nurse's aides provide services prescribed by the patient's physician. Intermediate-care facilities (ICF), sometimes called health-related facilities (HRF), provide regular medical, nursing, social, and rehabilitative services in addition to room and board and are for people not fully capable of independent living but are ambulatory and able to participate in their own care.

The proportion of nursing homes certified as SNFs and ICFs varies from state to state, as do levels of care provided. Despite this, few differences have been found between the kinds of patients cared for in SNFs and ICFs in different states, and the Institute of Medicine Committee on Nursing Home Regulation (1986) recommended that the distinction between SNF and ICF should be dropped.

Foster-care or board-and-care programs provide a home for the patient in a smaller, more personalized setting. This type of facility differs widely from area to area, with some states licensing these facilities and some not. As in looking at any long-term-care facility, family members should ascertain that the potential caregivers and/or professional staff are able to meet the special needs of the Alzheimer patient.

Adult homes are usually more suitable for persons with mild to moderate memory loss. These homes may be privately owned, or they may be operated by voluntary or religious organizations. They provide a safe, structured, and social environment; however, only minimal supervision is provided. Therefore, residents must be able to take care of their own personal needs and get to a common dining room for meals.

If the patient is a veteran and there is a Veterans Administration (VA) hospital or nursing home in your area, this possibility should also be explored. It is often difficult to obtain a VA bed unless the patient has a service-connected disability; however, some VA hospitals have units for patients with AD and related dementing disorders, while other VA hospitals have their own nursing homes. It is worth the effort, though, since VA services may be available for no fee or on a sliding scale. If your family is a member of an organization that sponsors a nursing home, such as the Knights of Columbus or a religious group, contact them regarding available facilities.

Where to Start

Where do you start to find a residential-care facility? If the patient is in a hospital, the social worker there can help suggest several that might be suitable. If, as in most cases, the patient is at home, you can seek the help of your family physician, clergy, County Department of Social Services, local ADRDA chapter, family and mental-health agencies, or other resources in your area. If possible, you should try to speak with others who have had experiences with nearby facilities, but keep in mind that different patients may require different types of care. Some may wander and will need a protected facility to prevent them from getting lost; others may need a great deal of assistance with toileting, dressing, and eating but may not wander. Make a list of what is most important and arrange appointments to visit each site. What is important for the Alzheimer patient and what is important for the caregiver may differ somewhat in that as a caregiver you will be much more aware of the physical surroundings. But it's very important that you select a place that you will be comfortable visiting.

Choosing a Facility

When choosing a long-term-care facility, what are you looking for and what questions should you ask? First of all, try to have another family member or a friend go with you to look at the facility. If you have never been to a long-term-care facility before, this may be very traumatic, and it is a comfort to have someone accompany you.

First, the facility should be clean, cheerful, and free of unpleasant odors. It must be easily accessible so that visiting is convenient for family and friends. The patient may not be aware of the environment, but the family that makes frequent visits will be. Furthermore, you should observe the following: Does the staff appear warm, friendly, and caring? Are the residents kept clean and neat? Are the majority of residents out of bed and dressed? Is there an activities schedule? Are the patients engaged in organized activities, or are they usually staring blankly at a television set? Are there provisions for the special needs of the demented patients? What is the ratio of staff to residents? Is the food attractively served? Are dietary requirements catered to? Is there adequate help provided with the mechanics of eating—unwrapping bread, opening milk containers, cutting meat, etc.?

Second, it is important to discuss fully the financial aspect with the administrator or admissions director. Charges vary with each facility, and it is best to know your obligations in advance so that you can make your decisions accordingly. When the bill arrives, you do not want any surprises or misunderstandings. If the rate is not all-inclusive, ask for a copy of the facility's rate chart to ascertain what additional charges you will be billed for, for example, medications, diapers, and laundry. In addition, make sure the nursing home will accept Medicaid reimbursement if and when the patient's private funds are exhausted.

If the patient is to be placed in an intermediate-care facility (ICF or HRF), it is also important to check on the procedure for transfer to a higher level of care if and when it becomes necessary. In some facilities, this transfer may be automatic, depending on the availability of an open bed. In others, the family may need to reapply or apply to another facility with an advanced level of care (SNF). This is especially true if the chosen facility does not have multiple levels of care.

Moving In

You have weighed your options and finally made your choice. The agony of making the decision is over. It is now time to try to explain to your loved one as simply as possible where he is going. He may or may not understand, but he will probably be aware of all the unfamiliar faces that confront him upon arrival at the facility. Assure him that you will be visiting frequently and that you are not far away if he needs you. Emphasize the positive aspects, the entertainment or various other activities that will be available for his enjoyment. If he can no longer participate in such activities, just knowing that you will be visiting often will reassure him.

Gather together family photographs, a plant, or special mementos that might hold meaning for your loved one and take them with you to the facility. It will be important for the patient to have familiar objects around him, giving the room a more personal feeling not only for the resident but also for the family and friends who visit.

The facility will advise you of the type of clothing and what personal items you should bring on the day of admission. Don't feel that you need to bring everything at once, for you can always bring additional clothes or toilet items on your next visit.

These first days of separation will not be easy for the caregiver. You will feel relief and guilt. You will be happy that a burden has been lifted from your shoulders but also uneasy that you are walking out of the facility and your loved one is staying—probably never to return home. You will need the comfort and support of good friends and family to help you over these lonely and difficult days. But remind yourself over and over again that trained professionals will care for your loved one. Frequent visits will satisfy you that he is well fed, clean, and reasonably happy.

Visiting

Those people who are important to the patient should arrange a schedule to share visitations. It is far better to spread out the visits than for everyone to come on the same day, for it not only is less confusing for the Alzheimer patient but will also spread out the joy of the visits. I found that planning my visits at mealtimes gave them more meaning. I could feed my husband and share a meaningful experience with him, since he no longer was able to talk. My husband loved ice cream, and the staff would provide ice cream so I could feed him something I knew he enjoyed. In addition, they would send a tray of food for me to his room, and we would eat together. I was made to feel that this was also my home, and I will always be grateful for their kindness to me. It should be noted that some facilities may be more flexible in this regard than others. Some may even discourage visiting at mealtimes. It's best to ask questions about visiting policies before you decide on a given facility.

Keeping in Touch

The staff should know that you are deeply concerned about the care that is given. Share with them little hints that you have learned in handling your patient and let them know what you expect. For example, I requested that my husband be bathed and shaved daily, although showers were not required to be given daily.

It was important to me that I see my husband almost every day. Fortunately, I was able to do this, but not all family members have the time because of other obligations. I would vary the time of my visits so that I could meet the staff on different shifts. Many caregivers may choose to visit far less frequently, perhaps weekly, as they simultaneously try to rebuild their own lives. Telephone contact may be maintained with the nursing or social-work staff between visits.

Try to develop a good rapport with the floor nurse and discuss the condition of the patient with her or him so that you will be aware of any new developments in your loved one's condition. If you are dissatisfied with the care, speak with the floor nurse first about your complaints.

In an SNF, patients must be seen monthly by a physician,

and it is a good practice to keep in touch with the doctor. Your physician and the facility should be advised of what heroic measures you do or do *not* wish to be taken in case a life-threatening crisis should arise. If the family wishes an autopsy performed after death, this information should be written on the patient's chart, with clear instructions, including the name and telephone numbers of the person(s) to be contacted regarding this procedure.

Once you have placed your loved one in a facility, try to be realistic and honest with yourself. AD is an insidious, degenerative disorder. To date, there is no cure. Don't expect your loved one to recover. Some days will be better than others, but be content that your patient is in a protective environment and is being cared for by people who understand his condition and know how to deal with it. You, the caregiver, will now be able to do many of the things that you were unable to do before, and now is the time to try to rebuild your own life.

In summary, placement of a loved one in a facility requires the whole family to make new adjustments and to develop new ways of coping. Good friends and other social supports may ease the way through a very difficult time. This period can also become a time of growth, when you as a caregiver can use your personal capacities and inner resources to face new challenges and confront new options for living your own life.

Glossary

SNF skilled nursing facilities provide continuous nursing care around the clock for convalescent or chronically ill patients.

ICF (HRF) intermediate-care facilities, sometimes called health-related facilities, provide regular medical, nursing, social, and rehabilitative services in addition to room and board and are for people who are not fully capable of independent living.

References

Lincoln, E., ed. 1980. *Choosing a nursing home for the person with intellectual loss*. Booklet prepared by the Burke Rehabilitation Center, White Plains, N.Y.

Mace, N. L., and Rabins, P. V. 1981. Nursing homes and other living arrangements. In *The 36-hour day: a family guide to caring for persons with Alzheimer's disease, related dementing illnesses, and memory loss in later life*. Baltimore: The Johns Hopkins University Press. (Available through ADRDA)

CHAPTER SIXTEEN

Nursing-Home-Care Issues

Lisa P. Gwyther, M.S.W.

NURSING-HOME PLACEMENT is perhaps the most difficult decision for a family coping with Alzheimer's disease (AD). When should a family consider it? What should you know about nursing homes before looking for a suitable facility? Are there systematic ways to evaluate facilities? Do the patient, family, and staff experience predictable reactions to admission? Are there special requirements for nursing-home care of AD patients and their families? Are these special requirements better met in specialized facilities? Can the quality of family visits improve during a long nursing-home stay? What about terminal care in nursing homes? This chapter will address these and other questions faced by many families caring for relatives with AD.

Nursing-Home Care

About twenty-two thousand nursing homes care for 1.1 million older Americans, providing care that ranges from excellent to abysmal.* While 80 percent of nursing homes are in business for profit, one cannot assume that nonprofit or philanthropic homes necessarily provide better care. At best, philanthropics have organized communities to raise funds, encourage professionalism, or enrich cultural or religious programming. Some public facilities, such as Veterans Administration (VA) hospitals, have excellent nursing-home units, but these are not necessarily readily accessible. Political clout is often required to gain admission for a patient with a non-service-connected disability such as AD.

There are various levels of residential/institutional care, and the names of these levels may vary among states. In general, nursing homes offer intermediate or skilled levels of care. A 1986 Institute of Medicine report recommended abolishing these arbitrary levels of care. These categories are based on minimal staffing levels. Often they do not adequately reflect the range of skills or services necessary for effective care.

Financing nursing-home care is a complex process. Medicaid pays for almost half of all nursing-home care, but a patient must practically impoverish himself or herself and sometimes a well spouse before becoming eligible for this program. Medicare and private health insurance pay almost nothing. Most families learn that they must save enough money to permit the patient to enter a nursing home as a private patient—paying the nursing home before becoming eligible for Medicaid by "spending down" (see chapters 18 and 19).

Today, nursing homes face incredible challenges. Many older people with acute problems are being discharged from hospitals to nursing homes much earlier and in a much sicker condition. These people may need a brief period of highly skilled hospitallike care. On the other hand, AD patients (who probably represent 60 percent of the total nursing-home population) need a dignified place to live and receive in-

Wall Street Journal, 11 February 1985.

creasing amounts of personal care and appropriate treatment for occasional acute illness. AD patients make heavy
demands on limited nursing-aide time. Also, their unpredictable behavior and lack of impulse control can be fright-
ening to aides, who must be constantly vigilant, and to other
frail patients, who may feel threatened by the AD patient's
vigor.

What families want from a facility varies as much as individual families do. Nursing homes also face constantly
changing regulations, increasing paperwork, and more vo-
cal, demanding communities. Families of nursing-home patients are demanding more personal-care nursing time per
patient, less reliance on chemical or physical restraints, and
more attention to quality-of-life issues. In this frustrating and
complex relationship among patients, families, providers,
and reimbursement sources, there are no consistent guidelines, standards, or expectations.

When Should a Family Consider Placement?

There is no right time for an AD patient to move to a nursing facility. Having AD means that a person will become
more dependent for personal care and supervision over time,
but the great variability observed among AD patients pre-
cludes the possibility of hard-and-fast guidelines for timing
placement. Earlier in the course of the disease, families may
have found it similarly difficult to determine when the patient could no longer be left alone safely. All such decisions
usually involve choices among equally unattractive options.

The AD patient's loss of adult reasoning and judgment
excludes his or her involvement in the placement decision.
Family members are often forced to make this difficult decision when they are physically, emotionally, or financially
exhausted. To make matters worse, the patient may be extremely angry, suspicious, and frightened at the prospect of

abandonment. "Love is doing what people need—not just what they want."* These words sound reassuring until you are walking out of a nursing home, leaving behind a parent or spouse who does not want to be there. It is easy to think this placement means you've abandoned your family member.

Families often turn to professionals, especially physicians, for help in determining when and where to place the patient. The physician's continuing care may be important to the family, and a physician's assessment and referral are usually required for admission. Even more important, the physician's authority and expertise can reassure the family, helping them reach the consensus that they have done their best for as long as possible. A physician can be most helpful if he or she is familiar with AD care and with both the patient and family situation. Families may also seek assistance from other qualified professionals, such as social workers, nurses, and gerontologists.

Unfortunately, in many cases decisions about placement are made hastily at a time of crisis by one family member, who may assume that there is no time to evaluate options or facilities or to consult relatives who live at a distance. The risks inherent in these crisis-time decisions may include several dislocating moves for the patient or sabotage of the placement by relatives who were not initially consulted.

What Predicts Placement?

If there is no right time for nursing-home care, what predicts the actual placement of an AD patient? Money is a significant predictor. Families with financial resources have more options in selecting appropriate facilities or services. Most families recognize that they cannot afford prolonged institutional care and therefore put it off for as long as possible,

*Manning 1984.

sometimes to the detriment of the primary caregiver's health. Many patients who could benefit from nursing-home care have too few funds to pay privately and too much income to qualify for Medicaid assistance and thus may not ever enter a nursing home.

Some families resist placement because it conflicts with cultural, religious, or family expectations or promises. Some families can't accept any group situation because it doesn't offer the personalized care available at home. Others distrust nursing homes because of media sensationalism, memories of unpleasant visits to inadequate facilities, or realistic observations that nursing homes have their limitations. These factors may prevent placement from ever occurring or may postpone placement until a crisis situation occurs. Family caregivers often cite specific stressful events or "last straws" that encouraged them to make the placement decision.

The time of placement is also influenced by the variability among family caregivers in their capacities to tolerate the stresses of caregiving. Spouses may expect to care for each other in a final illness, but older spousal caregivers may have to relinquish physical care due to frailty, chronic illness, or emotional exhaustion. Older wives face special problems if their physical size and strength are inadequate to manage a larger husband who is immobile or violent.

Adult children are more likely to seek placement for the patient, as they may be emotionally unprepared to care for a surviving parent. An adult child's life-style is rarely flexible enough to assume continuous responsibility for a parent. Many adults feel uncomfortable bathing a resistant but once powerful or attractive parent. Some families can't provide the constant care needed by a patient who has bedsores or is incontinent.

Moreover, there are other selection factors. There are marked regional differences in the availability of nursing-home beds. The most available beds are in the southwestern United States, and the least are in the Southeast. Highly regarded nursing homes with long waiting lists may select easier care—or private pay—patients when a rare opening exists. Because three-quarters of nursing-home patients are women, only one out of four available beds is open to a man.

Questions to Ask

It's helpful for a family to ask the following questions regarding placement:

1. Would the patient recognize a change in environment?
2. Does the patient recognize family members separate from the care provider?
3. Is the care needed beyond the family caregiver's capacity?
4. Might the patient unintentionally harm himself or others?
5. Would more stimulating activities and peer support benefit the patient?

The right time for placement is a family decision, hopefully made with the best available professional support and advice. The decision should reflect careful consideration of the needs of all generations within the family. While the placement should be made when the time seems right, preparation for eventual nursing-home care should be made well in advance.

How to Evaluate Facilities

Start with comprehensive patient and family assessment and counseling from a health professional or family agency. These should uncover "excess disabilities"; that is, coexisting treatable conditions, if there are any, determine the current and projected level of care needed by the patient and help establish a mutually agreeable plan for care. Next, an assessment of the patient's finances will determine the type of facility he or she can afford. Remember to consider how payment of nursing-home costs will affect a surviving spouse and be sure to ask about all extra costs. If a contract is involved, seek legal consultation.

Next, select a geographic area accessible to the most cherished and available visitors, including clergy and the primary-care physician if he or she will provide medical supervision once the patient enters the facility. Collect information about facilities from friends, trusted professionals, nursing-home advocacy organizations, the local nursing-home ombudsman, and most important, from members of ADRDA chapters and support groups. ADRDA families are probably the best critics of available facilities. Local and state regulatory agencies keep lists of deficiencies cited at local licensed homes, and some maintain lists of available beds. Aging agencies and county social-service departments may be good sources of information, as well.

The first look at a prospective home for someone you love can be overwhelming. A scheduled first visit usually includes a tour of the facility with an administrator, nurse, or social worker, who can respond to the questions on your list. Allow time to talk with residents and visitors, observe a meal and compare it to the posted menu, and notice the interaction of aides caring for residents. Take a checklist to evaluate the facility's strengths and weaknesses systematically and use it later to compare facilities.

Ask to see all areas of the facility, including the kitchen and bathing areas. Look at the overall pleasantness of the environment. Tour with your eyes, ears, and nose. Strong urine odors and heavy chemical scents should raise suspicion. Check temperatures and lighting. Are the patients up and around? AD patients function better when they are up and dressed in comfortable, familiar clothes each day and when they are treated with respect and warmth by staff and visitors.

Ask about staffing. Make sure the facility has a registered nurse (RN) or licensed practical nurse (LPN) on each shift. Some studies indicate that the proportion of registered-nurse hours per patient is directly related to the quality of patient care. No matter what the proportion of registered-nurse hours, most of the hands-on care is generally provided by nurse's aides, so it is wise to observe their interaction with patients. Does the direct-care staff handle patients gently? Do they speak directly *to* the patients or *about* them? Are they expected to do housekeeping and laundry as well as patient care? How many patients are assigned to each aide?

A nursing home's food-service expenditure also reflects the quality of care. Check the quality and quantity of food, attention to special diets, as well as available assistance for patients who can't feed themselves. Ask also about whether snacks are available between meals and how the staff encourages adequate fluid intake.

Ask about policies on safety, emergencies, wandering, fires, personal possessions, visiting hours, and use of physical or chemical restraints. Ask what will happen to a private-pay patient when he or she must apply for Medicaid. Ask about staff turnover. A consistent and familiar staff are important to the security of AD patients and their families.

Finally, check the degree of personalization offered by the facility. Can you differentiate residents and rooms on the basis of personal mementos and belongings? Does the facility encourage family involvement in care? Do the available activities help the patient maintain function and self-esteem?

You might wish to follow up with one or two unannounced visits at various times of the day and evening. Remember that shiny new hospitallike environments may be more pleasing to visitors than they are comfortable for AD patients. A warm atmosphere and interaction among residents, staff, and visitors may be much more conducive to overall quality of life.

The checklist at the end of this chapter will help you evaluate a prospective nursing home.

Adjustment to Admission

It's scary for anyone who is confused to face new people, surroundings, and routines. The "typical" AD patient may feel abandoned, lost, or "tricked" upon admission, and he or she may be angry, suspicious, withdrawn, agitated, or afraid. Often the patient frantically searches the halls and other people's rooms or possessions for something familiar. The patient's distorted sense of time may make it impossible for him or her to know when it's mealtime and whether or not he or she has eaten. Loss of impulse control and learned polite behavior may mean the patient will eat sloppily, stuff food in a pocket, disrobe in public, or mistakenly feel attacked by an aide who is trying to help with bathing or dressing. It helps to stay close, assist the staff in understanding the patient's routine, and gently answer the patient's frantic questions. Routine escort saves the patient from getting lost or being embarrassed at not finding the bathroom.

On the other hand, some patients go through a "honeymoon" phase on admission, responding positively to a structured routine. AD patients often "improve" when they leave a home they thought wasn't their "real" home. Even better, they may feel relieved of the pressure to remain "head of household."

Staff, roommates, and other residents need time to adjust to a new AD resident. Experienced staff members learn to withhold judgment about an AD patient's needs based only on the first day's observation. AD patients need time to recover from the relocation and to regain remaining function with proper assistance. Family members can help the staff understand who this patient was before the illness and how best to respond to his or her present needs. Sharing parts of the patient's history helps the staff individualize care and thereby also makes their work more interesting.

Beware of any facility that insists the family leave the patient alone for the first few weeks. This "boot camp" approach to adjustment further frightens patients, exacerbates family helplessness, and shows no respect for patient or family feelings.

Specialized Nursing Homes/Units: Pros and Cons

A definition of "best" care awaits our better understanding of AD. Innovations are needed, but no single setting or therapeutic strategy will be ideal for such a heterogeneous group of patients. The focus on improving care limits adversarial relationships between families and providers, and model programs may serve to expand the creative potential of *all* levels of staff. The challenge of special care is in resolving potential conflicts among safety, aesthetics, cost, and regulations, and what pleases one group of people may offend another. For example, one family found their grandmother was easily comforted by an old rag doll she had had years earlier and saw to it that the doll stayed with the grandmother in her care facility. They later were disturbed to learn that state surveyors cited their grandmother's facility for "demeaning" treatment of adults (i.e., allowing her to have a toy).

Some special-care units have been described as "offering sheltered freedom." These units are generally small and more manageable communities of AD patients who are still able to give and receive support from each other as well as from staff, family, and visitors. These units serve very few people. Each unit may serve a maximum of fifteen patients. Most of these units are experimental and not available in most communities. In general, the more restless, moderately impaired patient may benefit most from the expanded energy outlets and structured programming available in other special units. The environment permits care that may not be possible in larger settings.

While it may be too early to set standards or guidelines for special-care units, one can make some educated guesses about ideal facilities of the future. They will probably be smaller (units of larger facilities offering a broader range of care levels) and homier, with safer benign environments allowing patients more freedom under continuous staff observation. Each unit will accommodate ten to twenty patients. Inviting indoor and outdoor recreation areas could offer places to work off excess energy. Disoriented residents could have meaningful personal objects nearby to help them identify their space, a practice presently discouraged to avoid loss, theft, or damage. Toilets in plain view with frequent reminders to use them may cue patient associations. Individualized activity plans could be based on past *and* present interests to include productive work roles and opportunities for socialization.

In summary, placement in special-care units should be based on the individual patient's capacity to benefit from special programming. These units may therefore have limited applicability. The course of AD changes over time, and so, too, do the needs for care. Eventually, patients require the skilled nursing care that is available in most combined ICF/SNF facilities. AD patients may also have other concurrent illnesses or disabilities, requiring a broader spectrum of services than those offered in specialized units.

As a family, you should ask what is "special" in any nursing home that markets a special unit, Alzheimer facility, or program. Be wary of any "special" program that does not significantly differ from a traditional nursing home in size, environment, activities, personal care, safety, or staffing. If the only difference in the special versus traditional facility is cost and diagnostic segregation, look elsewhere. If the wing or unit serves only patients at a specific stage of dementing illness, what will happen when your relative's illness progresses? What about other illnesses or disabilities that may afflict the patient in a special unit? If, for example, the unit serves only ambulatory patients or offers only intermediate-level care, what happens to the patient who falls and requires special therapy following a hip fracture? As with any facility, you should ask about special costs or fees associated with the program. Currently, many special-care units are entirely private pay. If this is the case, will the patient be moved off the unit when his or her assets run out? Some special units charge more than the current skilled-nursing-home rate in a local area. While this may be justified on the basis of increased staff costs, the facility should be held accountable for its rates.

Managing Behavioral Symptoms

Coping with behavioral symptoms of dementia challenges even the most experienced nursing-home staff, but there are suggested strategies for coping with AD patients' problem behaviors. For example, it is probably best to adapt staff responses and environment to patients rather than requiring vulnerable patients to adapt to nursing-home rules. Staff members can change their behavior more readily and in less time. A broad use of such indirect strategies throughout a facility offers positive results for all patients whether in special or integrated units.

Visiting

Families of recently admitted nursing-home patients are perhaps more stressed than at other points in the disease process. Emotional responsibility for an AD relative isn't relieved just because one is relieved of physical care. Often family stress is heightened at this point because of conflict about the appropriateness of placement. This is a time when family caregivers may be more isolated than ever and a time when they need the greatest amount of family and social support.

For many couples it's important to be together regardless of the AD patient's recognition of the spouse. Many spousal caregivers follow the patient to the facility, initially spending almost as much time with the patient as they did at home. Gradually, these families come to trust the staff and may begin to let go. However, rebuilding a single life for a surviving spouse outside the facility takes time.

Other family members may find nursing-home visits too uncomfortable, preferring to "remember the patient as he or she was." This further isolates the lone-spouse visitor from needed support, although many spouses try to be understanding about their children's reluctance to visit. Most family members, however, want to continue some meaningful role in patient care, whether it's helping the patient with eating, doing laundry, taking walks, or just sharing moments of personal affection.

When visiting, it is important to keep in mind that for many staff members, the rewards of work come from working with families who can appreciate their efforts and share their frustration with a disease that worsens despite the best care. Staff members appreciate families who are open to and with them, retain a sense of humor, and recognize them as individuals apart from their duties at the facility. For example, an aide may work with several patients, all of whom are incapable of asking about her new baby, but she may appreciate such concern expressed by regular family visitors. It's important for you to establish close contact with the staff caring for your loved one; patient, family, and staff will all benefit from this increased concern.

The Long Haul: Making Visits Count

Once a patient settles into the nursing home, families must redefine their relationships with their impaired relative and are forced to acknowledge that relationships are not as they would wish. Nonetheless, visits *do* count. Family visits offer nursing-home patients invaluable personal attention, affection, dignity, recognition, and a feeling of continuity.

Old patterns of family visiting don't work in the new setting of the care facility, and you should be prepared for the conversation to change drastically. Family events that were important to the patient before, such as the activities of grandchildren or a business, may no longer capture his or her attention. Creativity is essential to break through the barrier of impaired adult thinking and memory. Preparing and serving a favorite or traditional food, decorating the patient's room for a holiday, giving the patient a manicure, new hairdo, or beauty treatment, or just reminiscing over old scrapbooks or pictures, may enhance the quality of time spent visiting together.

"Will you take me home?"
I cannot take you home.
But I can comfort you when the floor shimmers like a
    sunlit lake.
I can wait while you layer, like memories, tissue precisely
    on tissue
And remember for you who you are and what you have
    done.
I can give you order and refuge in the strange land you
    inhabit now.
I can love you as you are,

. . . .

But my hand cannot remold (such a fragile piece as you).
No, I wish, but I cannot take you home.

ELIZABETH MANDLEN
ADRDA Baltimore *Newsletter*, Fall 1985

When a loved one is placed in a facility, a well spouse must learn to live with an overwhelming sense of loss—loss of identity (a married person in limbo, in relation to his or her social position), loss of purpose (after days were filled with work or care of the patient), and loss of that part of oneself that becomes tied to a long-term marital partner. Most AD families are forced to be good problem solvers but may find it easier to mobilize for the short haul than to settle in for a long period of "coping" after a loved one enters a facility. Good friends can buffer the losses experienced when institutionalization leaves a well spouse alone at home. If you're that well spouse, you should rely on these good friends to help you ease the loneliness of your spouse's absence as well as to visit your loved one in your absence or to check on him or her if you are ill.

Coping successfully with an AD relative at any stage is usually summarized by families with some phrase like "I get by with a sense of humor, good friends, the grace of God, and old-fashioned ingenuity." These intuitive coping strategies work well for families of institutionalized dementia patients. Visits to the facility force one to develop or refine a sense of humor and build tolerance for the patient's mental confusion. Pleasure in the moment becomes a reasonable visiting goal.

A strong religious faith helps many families withstand the bad things happening to them. Some persons find that sharing moments of silent prayer, attending chapel services in the nursing home, visiting with clergy, reading Bible stories, or singing hymns from childhood enrich the time spent together.

Relatives and friends should spread out visits, arriving one or two at a time, to provide personal attention and stimulation in manageable doses. Brief, frequent visits work best. Because AD patients are so sensitive to nonverbal cues, it's best not to squeeze in visits when pressed for time. The patient may respond to your hurried appearance with agitation or withdrawal, leaving both of you frustrated. Conversely, some patients find one-on-one attention too demanding. It may also be wise to get to know other residents and their families. Small groups can dilute the intensity of visits, and regular visitors can cover for each other when on vacation.

A wise family visitor becomes part of the patient's familiar routine. Regular visitors can encourage their relatives to participate in activities by attending parties or by helping them create small social groups. For example, if the patient was used to visiting over a card game or coffee, a small group could be set up around this familiar activity.

Writing out family information for the staff on all three shifts of duty may assure your relative of more consistent care. One daughter created an elegant, framed, old-fashioned sampler that she hung over her silent mother's bed. In several cross-stitched lines, she described her mother and how she would like to be treated. The staff and other family visitors were so impressed that many replicas later appeared. The mother also loved hearing about her daughter's skill in creating the gift for her.

AD patients may have sudden, inexplicable mood changes. Often they can't explain why they are crying, frightened, or angry, but they may appreciate a visitor who stays close by, hugs, or just holds him or her until the bad feeling disappears. Reminding the AD patient to concentrate on positive features may be another strategy to help alleviate the bad mood. A family visitor who comments on the patient's gorgeous thick hair, dancing eyes, or athletic build can still bring pleasure to someone who doesn't even recognize who is speaking.

As a family member who visits regularly, you will doubtless experience a day when the patient seems unusually lucid or in rare high spirits. These moments of insight and recognition deserve celebration, but you should avoid making unrealistic assumptions about the patient's recovery. In some of these insightful moments, the patient's old sense of humor may come through. An AD patient recently admitted to a special-care unit was moping around and obviously sad. A visitor to another patient commented on his beautiful tan and asked him if he'd been on a cruise recently. He looked up with interest for the first time and said clearly, "Baby, this ain't no cruise!"

Some facilities encourage families to bring in visitor logs, photo albums, or scrapbooks to look at during visits. Guest books remind the patient of those friends who care and visit, and AD patients generally talk more meaningfully about pictures and events from the past. Stories may be repeated often, but the pleasure in the retelling is an end in itself.

Terminal Care

There comes a point in dementing illness when the patient ultimately withdraws. Perhaps he or she may sleep more, become immobile, or lose interest in food, drink, and previously pleasurable activities. It's difficult to know at this point what the patient is thinking or wanting, and families once again face lonely ethical dilemmas.

Families should make their wishes for terminal care known to the medical and nursing staff. It is usually helpful to learn about the options and consequences of different treatment courses. (This is discussed in chapter 20 of this book.) The physician will probably request family guidance on feeding, hospitalization, treatment of infections, and autopsy. One has to assume that the patient trusts the family to act compassionately in his or her behalf.

Terminal care involves skilled nursing, with particular attention to hydration, nutrition, cleanliness, skin condition, and comfortable positioning. Concern for dignity and comfort becomes prominent in the terminal phase. The family will want the patient repositioned frequently and adequately nourished to prevent skin breakdown. Fluids become more essential than food if the patient isn't moving enough to burn calories. Range-of-motion exercises may limit contractures, and prevention of falls, which are often terminal events for AD patients, takes on greater significance.

Even if the AD patient isn't communicative, the closeness and intimacy of continuing visits are important. Visits may be spent combing the patient's hair, rubbing his or her skin with a moisturizer, listening to music or religious services together, or sitting outdoors. Some family visitors initiate one-way conversations with hopes that the feeling tone, if not the words, will get through. This is a time when conflicted family relationships may be more easily resolved. Everyone may be feeling more forgiving and compassionate, and time together takes on a special significance.

Regardless of how prepared a family feels for the loss of the patient, death may come unexpectedly. It's best to anticipate and plan for all possible scenarios, making sure all concerned family and staff understand your wishes. Most families who have been involved with the patient throughout the illness are even more surprised at how unprepared they are for their reactions to the death. Their strength often comes from their confidence that they honored their commitment throughout the illness.

Hope for the Future

Biomedical research offers much hope for future prevention, treatment, and cure of dementing illness. However, today's hope rests on continued research on residential care. The demand for quality nursing-home care at a bearable cost will continue to escalate as American family trees become increasingly top-heavy and more older people become dependent for chronic care on fewer available relatives. Nursing homes are coming into the mainstream of health care, and with it some form of long-term-care insurance *coverage* will become essential. Currently, we have no long-term health-care policy and no long-term care "system." What exists is a complex patchwork of diverse services, of uneven quality, poorly coordinated, and unevenly distributed. This nonsystem doesn't work for complex long-term problems such as AD. Our major health-care reimbursement programs, Medicare and Medicaid, are not meeting public expectations. Medicare is not paying for nursing-home care, and it probably never will. Medicaid eligibility for nursing-home care often represents the impoverishment of both poor and middle-income families.

While optimal models are not obvious, we do have examples of successful residential/institutional programs that report positive outcomes. As more model programs are tested over time, more reasonable demands can be made for quality assurance, standards, regulations, and enforcement. In the meantime, families must continue to honor their commitment to institutionalized relatives by advocating improved quality of care.

The Visit

It isn't much, it's only a smile,
Never a lot, just once in a while.
What does it mean? Who's to say?
All I know is . . . it made my day.

The face so handsome as of yore,
The stately stance, now no more,
Yet serene in a placid way,
Still beautiful to me . . . it made my day.

Know me? A fleeting "yes."
My hug and kiss I must confess
Was returned to me the same way.
It felt so good . . . it made my day.

It isn't much, it's only a smile,
Never a lot, just once in a while.
What does it mean? Who's to say?
All I know is . . . it made my day.

T. F. RITTENBERG
ADRDA Denver *Newsletter*, Spring 1986

References

Gwyther, L. 1985. *Care of Alzheimer patients: a manual for nursing home staff.* American Health Care Association and Alzheimer's Disease and Related Disorders Association. (Available through ADRDA)

———. May 1986. Treating behavior as a symptom of illness. *The Provider.*

Manning, D. 1984. *When love gets tough: the nursing home decision.* Hereford, Texas: Insite Press.

Nursing-Home Checklist

	Yes	No
1. Does the home have a current license from the state?	___	___
2. Does the administrator have a current license from the state?	___	___
3. If you need and are eligible for financial assistance, is the home certified to participate in government or other programs that provide it?	___	___
4. Does the home provide special services such as a specific diet or therapy that the patient needs?	___	___

PHYSICAL CONSIDERATIONS

	Yes	No
5. Location		
a. Pleasing to the patients?	___	___
b. Convenient for patient's personal doctor?	___	___

    c. Convenient for frequent visits?   ___ ___
    d. Near a hospital?   ___ ___

6. Accident prevention
    a. Well lighted inside?   ___ ___
    b. Free of hazards underfoot?   ___ ___
    c. Chairs sturdy and not easily tipped?   ___ ___
    d. Warning signs posted around freshly
       waxed floors?   ___ ___
    e. Handrails in hallways and grab bars in
       bathroom?   ___ ___

7. Fire safety
    a. Meets federal and/or state codes?   ___ ___
    b. Exits clearly marked and unobstructed?   ___ ___
    c. Written emergency-evacuation plan?   ___ ___
    d. Frequent fire drills?   ___ ___
    e. Exit doors not locked on the inside?   ___ ___
    f. Stairways enclosed and doors to stairways
      kept closed?   ___ ___

8. Bedrooms
    a. Open on to hall?   ___ ___
    b. Window?   ___ ___
    c. No more than four beds per room?   ___ ___
    d. Easy access to each bed?   ___ ___
    e. Drapery for each bed?   ___ ___
    f. Nurse call bell by each bed?   ___ ___
    g. Fresh drinking water at each bed?   ___ ___
    h. At least one comfortable chair per patient?   ___ ___
    i. Reading lights?   ___ ___
    j. Clothes closet and drawers?   ___ ___
    k. Room for a wheelchair to maneuver?   ___ ___
    l. Care used in selecting roommates   ___ ___

9. Cleanliness
    a. Generally clean, even though it may have
       a lived-in look?   ___ ___
    b. Free of unpleasant odors?   ___ ___
    c. Incontinent patients given prompt atten-
       tion?   ___ ___

10. Lobby
    a. Is the atmosphere welcoming?   ___ ___
    b. If also a lounge, is it being used by resi-
       dents?   ___ ___

c. Furniture attractive and comfortable?   ___ ___
d. Plants and flowers?   ___ ___
e. Certificates and licenses on display?   ___ ___

11. Hallways
    a. Large enough for two wheelchairs to pass
       with ease?   ___ ___
    b. Hand-grip railing on the sides?   ___ ___

12. Dining room
    a. Attractive and inviting?   ___ ___
    b. Comfortable chairs and tables?   ___ ___
    c. Easy to move around in?   ___ ___
    d. Tables convenient for those in wheelchairs?   ___ ___
    e. Food tasty and attractively served?   ___ ___
    f. Meals match posted menu?   ___ ___
    g. Those needing help receiving it?   ___ ___

13. Kitchen
    a. Food preparation, dishwashing, and gar-
       bage areas separated?   ___ ___
    b. Food needing refrigeration not standing on
       counters?   ___ ___
    c. Kitchen help observe sanitation rules?   ___ ___

14. Activity rooms
    a. Rooms available for patients' activities?   ___ ___
    b. Equipment (such as games, easels, yarn,
       kiln, etc.) available?   ___ ___
    c. Residents using equipment?   ___ ___

15. Special-purpose rooms
    a. Rooms set aside for physical examinations
       or therapy?   ___ ___
    b. Rooms being used for stated purpose?   ___ ___

16. Isolation room
    a. At least one bed and bathroom available
       for patients with contagious illness?   ___ ___

17. Toilet facilities
    a. Convenient to bedrooms?   ___ ___
    b. Easy for a wheelchair patient to use?   ___ ___
    c. Sink?   ___ ___
    d. Nurse call bell?   ___ ___
    e. Hand grips on or near toilets?   ___ ___

f. Bathtubs and showers with nonslip surfaces? ___ ___

18. Grounds
    a. Residents can get fresh air? ___ ___
    b. Ramps to help handicapped? ___ ___

SERVICES

19. Medical
    a. Physician available in emergency? ___ ___
    b. Private physician allowed? ___ ___
    c. Regular medical attention assured? ___ ___
    d. Thorough physical immediately before or upon admission? ___ ___
    e. Medical records and plan of care kept? ___ ___
    f. Patient involved in developing plans for treatment? ___ ___
    g. Other medical services (dentists, optometrists, etc.) available regularly? ___ ___
    h. Freedom to purchase medicines outside home? ___ ___

20. Hospitalization
    a. Arrangement with nearby hospital for transfer when necessary? ___ ___

21. Nursing services
    a. RN responsible for nursing staff in a skilled nursing home? ___ ___
    b. LPN on duty day and night in a skilled nursing home? ___ ___
    c. Trained nurse's aides and orderlies on duty in homes providing some nursing care? ___ ___

22. Rehabilitation
    a. Specialists in various therapies available when needed? ___ ___

23. Activities program
    a. Individual patient preferences observed? ___ ___
    b. Group and individual activities? ___ ___
    c. Residents encouraged but not forced to participate? ___ ___

    d. Outside trips for those who can go?   —— ——
    e. Volunteers from the community work with
        patients?   —— ——

24. Religious observances
    a. Arrangements made for patient to worship
        as he or she pleases?   —— ——
    b. Religious observances a matter of choice?   —— ——

25. Social services
    a. Social worker available to help residents
        and families?   —— ——

26. Food
    a. Dietitian plans menus for patients on spe-
        cial diets?   —— ——
    b. Variety from meal to meal?   —— ——
    c. Meals served at normal times?   —— ——
    d. Plenty of time for each meal?   —— ——
    e. Snacks?   —— ——
    f. Food delivered to patients' rooms?   —— ——
    g. Help with eating given when needed?   —— ——

27. Grooming
    a. Barbers and beauticians available for men
        and women?   —— ——

ATTITUDES AND ATMOSPHERE

28. General atmosphere friendly and supportive?   —— ——

29. Residents retain human rights?
    a. May participate in planning treatment?   —— ——
    b. Medical records are held confidential?   —— ——
    c. Can veto experimental research?   —— ——
    d. Have freedom and privacy to attend to
        personal needs?   —— ——
    e. Married couples may share room?   —— ——
    f. All have opportunities to socialize?   —— ——
    g. May manage own finances if capable or ob-
        tain accounting if not?   —— ——
    h. May decorate their own bedrooms?   —— ——
    i. May wear their own clothes?   —— ——
    j. May communicate with anyone without
        censorship?   —— ——

262 H O W T O C O P E

k. Are not transferred or discharged arbitrar-
ily?   ____ ____

30. Administrator and staff available to discuss
problems?
   a. Patients and relatives can discuss complaints without fear of reprisal?   ____ ____
   b. Staff responds to calls quickly and cour-
teously?   ____ ____

31. Residents appear alert unless very ill?   ____ ____

32. Visiting hours accommodate residents and relatives?   ____ ____

33. Civil-rights regulations observed?   ____ ____

34. Visitors and volunteers pleased with home?   ____ ____

Scoring

Generally, the best home is the one for which you check the most
"yes" answers. However, different homes offer different services.
You must decide which services are most important to you.

If the answer to any of the first four questions is "no," do not use
the home.

PART III

Legal and Financial Aspects

CHAPTER SEVENTEEN

Ethical Dilemmas Facing Caregivers and Attorneys in Dealing with Legal, Financial, and Health-Care Decision Making

Nancy N. Dubler, LL.B., and
Peter J. Strauss, J.D.

THE PROBLEM OF INCREASING vulnerability to illness with advancing age has had a direct effect on the economic well-being of older persons. Because our national health-care system—the Medicare insurance program (supplemented, when affordable, by private health insurance)—is an acute-care system, it excludes coverage for preventive care, chronic care, long-term care, custodial care, most home care, and those personal and social services that could improve the health and well-being of many older Americans.

The United States is the only Western society with a health-care system that makes the distinction between acute care and chronic care. Since the elderly are more subject to chronic illness than acute illness, the health-care system in the United States essentially discriminates against them. Persons of modest means who develop expensive chronic illness such as Alzheimer's disease (AD) may thus be placed in the position of facing economic disaster in their retirement years. Ironically, the Medicaid program, a program designed for the poor, does extend to and cover many of the chronic- and custodial-care expenses that are excluded by Medicare, but to qualify for Medicaid assistance, a person must be "legally poor." As explained later in this section on legal issues, under the financial-eligibility rules, he or she must have nominal assets as a result of "spending down," or never having had assets, or "transferring" assets (by way of gift) at least two years prior to the time of application for Medicaid.

Confrontation with increasing levels of disability, with the uncertainty of access to health care and with the changing basis of federal reimbursement for care, is compounded by concerns about decision making for specific sorts of care in the future. Many older persons are concerned not only with access to new sorts of care but with their right to refuse such care in the future, especially if their decision-making abilities become diminished by illness.

Attorneys are increasingly consulted by older persons and their families to help them plan for the vagaries of illness and care in later life. More and more attorneys are being called upon to address financial-planning issues (wills, living trusts, durable power of attorney, estate planning, and arrangements for the transfer of assets) and health-care planning. Personal-care issues can be addressed by durable powers of attorney for health-care decisions and through the effective execution of living wills. The attorney must be knowledgeable about how the client's personal preference may be applied and extended beyond the time when the client may have lost the capacity to decide, so that medical technology will be applied in a manner that is consistent with personal desire.

Issues to Consider When Seeking Legal
Assistance: Who Is the Client?

An attorney may be contacted when the patient or the family anticipates problems with finances, benefit plans, or treatment decisions in the future. If it is the Alzheimer victim who contacts the attorney, outlines the issues, describes the disease process, and explains his or her goals for legal intervention and future care, the attorney is faced with no particular illness-specific problem. Attorney and client then work together to identify and address those issues that presently exist or may arise in the future. This scenario would be limited to early cases of AD.

In most instances involving AD, it is not the patient who contacts the attorney but a member of that person's family. In these cases, because of the nature of some of the strategies that must be employed, there is the possibility that the rights of the patient and those of the patient's spouse or children may be in conflict. The family member needs to be aware that the attorney must decide, from the outset, who the client is. If the attorney determines that the client is the family member rather than the patient, then a number of questions arise:

1. What is the attorney's obligation to assure adequate legal representation for the patient?
2. Does the obligation to ensure legal representation exist only if the needs of patient and family are in conflict or in any event?
3. Are the legal steps appropriate in particular situations (such as transferring the patient's assets) in the best interest of the patient, the family member, or both? Who decides in the case of a conflict?
4. Could the attorney possibly conclude that all parties involved in the transaction are her clients despite any apparent or real conflicts?

5. Should the judgment of the attorney be affected by the existence of paranoid ideation in the patient that may accompany dementia?

In practice, the attorney is frequently called upon to make ethical and moral judgments concerning issues that are broader than strictly legal ones, such as motivation, family relationships, and the permissible range for surrogate proxy decisions. Does the attorney who makes these decisions take on the functions of the court? Are these decisions beyond the lawyer's abilities as a professional and responsibilities as an officer of the court?

Although there may be no answers at present, these are questions that the family of an Alzheimer patient should keep in mind when seeking legal advice.

In many cases, for example, the patient is the owner of a substantial portion of the family assets, and the spouse can be impoverished by the costs of health care if all of these assets are to be "spent down" on the patient's care before Medicaid becomes available. Here the spouse needs protection—but so does the patient. When appropriate, transferring assets to the healthy spouse will protect both the patient and the spouse. It is in the patient's interest to preserve assets to pay for medical care, personal care, and living expenses that Medicaid will not cover. But questions arise: is this transfer of assets a benefit to the patient, or does such a plan result in a denial of the patient's rights?

THE PATIENT'S LEGAL CAPACITY

The family member who seeks legal advice later in the course of the illness may be told by the attorney that what appears to be the solution to the financial and legal problems of the patient and the family cannot be effectuated because of the patient's diminished capacity. Some understanding of what is meant by the term "legal capacity" will help the process of appropriate decision making.

The President's Commission for the Study of Ethical Problems in Medicine and Biomedical and Behavioral Research suggested that "decision-making capacity requires, to a greater or lesser degree: possession of a set of values and goals; the ability to communicate and to understand information; and the ability to reason and to deliberate about one's choices."

The definition of capacity, developed to meet the needs of a health-care system and to assure the adequacy of informed consent to medical care, may be directly applicable to the sorts of problems presented to an attorney. If the patient/client possesses sufficient capacity to participate in decision making, the issue of family involvement, or possible conflict, is largely eliminated. But who defines and determines legal capacity? And suppose the client does not have it?

Many definitions of capacity or competence are proposed in various statutes and judicial opinions. These definitions are often dependent on the context. For example, one may be "competent" to execute a will and not competent to enter a complex contract. Or one may be able to execute a contract and still be judged by the law as not capable of caring for minor children.

For the client capable of making decisions, the lawyer may recommend a range of options. Increasingly, living trusts and durable powers of attorney are being suggested to clients both for the effective management of assets beyond the onset of disability and for appropriate health advocacy in a situation in which the patient-client is no longer able to decide. All states (but not the District of Columbia) permit the execution of durable powers of attorney. Some states provide specifically that these delegations of authority may apply to health-care decisions, as well. The attorney may also assist the client in executing a living will. This document is an expression of the patient's desires in the event the patient cannot participate in decisions about care in the future. The effectiveness and the form vary from state to state. It is also highly recommended that a physician participate in the process to permit the greatest medical specificity. There is some question whether these documents will have effect outside the jurisdiction in which they are executed.

Clients who execute appropriate documents when capable of so doing protect themselves and their families from the uncertainty of a future confrontation with legal and ethical ambiguity and economic devastation. The lawyer who is called upon to assist the client in accomplishing these goals may face a dilemma: how to judge when a client no longer has the capacity to engage in this kind of planning and what to do if the lawyer believes the client cannot do so, even when such planning may be in the client's best interests. Thus, legal advice should be sought early in the illness.

Guardianship or Conservatorship

In recent years, states have enacted a form of limited guardianship or conservatorship. This exists in addition to the more traditional guardianship actions that require a judicial finding of incompetence. The humiliation of this designation and the panoply of rights that it destroys have led to a preference for less drastic and less restrictive interventions. Limited guardianships or conservatorships were designed to appoint individuals to manage the affairs and property of a person who, through the advance of disease or disability, has been rendered functionally incapable of doing so. In theory, most limited guardianships and conservatorships do not grant jurisdiction over the person. In fact, most statutes provide that the court designee not only deal with financial management but follow an approved personal-care plan. Therefore, to some extent finances do, in fact, determine personal-care choices.

This reality is most evident in regard to the issue of nursing-home placement. If the guardian or conservator has the power to expend money for the care of the patient and the patient is not competent to express his or her wishes, what obstacle is there to prevent implementation of the decision of the conservator to institutionalize the patient against his or her wishes? What procedures exist to ensure that a representative advocates for the views of the patient? In most states, no such mechanism exists.

The problem of advocacy for the wishes and rights of the patient who can no longer communicate his or her wishes arises in many contexts, including the basic conservatorship or guardianship proceeding itself. To initiate a conservatorship or guardianship proceeding, the family or other interested party must engage an attorney and petition the court. The statutes generally provide for the appointment of a guardian *ad litem* to represent the patient. Most statutes, however, are woefully unclear as to the role of the guardian *ad litem*. Does the guardian *ad litem* represent the present "spoken choice" of the patient, that is, the position articulated by the patient that may or may not reflect previous preference, present desire, and best interest, or does the guardian *ad litem* act as an independent fact finder for the court? If it is the latter and an independent judgment of what is the patient's best interest infuses the report of the guardian *ad litem*, then a major part of the adversary system is missing in the proceeding. What procedures do or should exist to ensure that a representative advocates for the position of the patient?

What is the obligation of an attorney who is called upon to represent the proposed ward as a guardian *ad litem* and is asked to advocate for the patient's viewpoint? What should that attorney do when he or she believes the "spoken choice" of the patient is not in the patient's best interest?

What is the obligation of a petitioning attorney to the proposed ward? Should that attorney be responsible for ensuring the presence of the proposed ward in the courtroom if the guardian *ad litem* has not so arranged? Should the attorney for the petitioner, knowing that the ward would desire to be present, bring that information to the attention of the court? Is it that attorney's obligation to advise the court about the wishes of the proposed ward that are in conflict with the position of the party bringing the proceeding if those views have not been adequately brought out in the hearing?

THE ISSUE OF PRIVILEGED COMMUNICATIONS

Involved in all of the foregoing issues is the issue of patient/physician privilege. When the attorney is dealing with planning for an incapacitated client, is the patient's physician permitted to disclose information regarding the client's mental or physical condition where the client cannot fully consent to the release of such information? What if the information will assist the attorney in developing a sensible and valid plan or in determining that the client does not have sufficient capacity?

In the context of a court proceeding for the appointment of a guardian or a conservator, can the physician be compelled to testify regarding the condition of the proposed incompetent over the objection of such person or without such person's consent? Can the physician's records and testimony be subpoenaed? Can the physician assist the attorney who represents the petitioner in preparing to proceed? Will this not interfere with the patient/physician privilege? Would such collusion be inconsistent with the attitude of the law toward protecting this privilege? On the other hand, the statutory procedures designed to provide assistance to incapacitated persons may well be emasculated without the ability to ascertain the facts. It may be that the appointment of a physician by the court to make an independent examination may be a solution in some cases but not in all. Court cases have not clearly resolved this problem, although there are decisions on both sides of the issue.

Confrontations with Health-Care Institutions: Patients' Rights

It is now settled in law and supported by bioethical theory that "every human being of adult years and sound mind has a right to determine what shall be done with his own body." This concept of self-determination, in conjunction with the constitutional right to privacy, supports the right of a patient to consent to or to refuse treatment. Who decides whether nasogastrointestinal feeding is to be instituted if the victim's family opposes it but the institution feels obligated to commence the procedure? The ability to conduct research with human subjects is constrained by federal regulation and infused by concepts of patients' rights. The issue is clear: the desire of society and the medical community to provide care and conduct scientific research often conflicts with the individual's right to refuse care and to refuse participation in experiments. This issue is further complicated in the case of the Alzheimer victim who no longer has the capacity to express his or her own view.

In jurisdictions in which the legal status of orders not to resuscitate is unclear, the family should determine whether a hospital follows a policy that is protective of the institution's interest and the patient's rights, or alternatively, does the hospital policy protect the interest of the institution even if a patient's rights are trampled in the process? Right-to-die issues are discussed further in the book.

Keep in mind that an attorney consulted about these issues is faced with serious ethical dilemmas. Again, the basic issue of representation must be resolved. Is the client the patient or the patient's family? Are the wishes of those parties clearly identifiable? Is the attorney an advocate for only the "spoken choice" of the patient, or does the attorney inject and advocate for his independent beliefs? How are the wishes of the family members incorporated?

Medicine has accommodated the graying of America by restructuring the doctor's office to permit elderly persons to maneuver without assistance and by inculcating skills in practitioners that include not only the usual diagnostic and treatment skills but knowledge about home care and benefit programs. In contrast, the law has just begun to recognize that elderly persons have specific needs for legal services and may be affected by disabilities that require varying approaches structurally and substantively in the law. The first textbooks and articles on law and the elderly have begun to appear, and a few law schools have introduced courses on legal problems of the elderly. Some government-funded legal-service programs for the elderly now exist, and a few attorneys are beginning to develop an expertise relevant to the problems of the elderly.

We have presented but a few of the ethical dilemmas faced by family members, attorneys, physicians, social workers, gerontologists, and other members of the health-care team. As AD progresses along its inevitable course, the decisions become more difficult and the traumas greater. Alzheimer families know this only too well.

Glossary

competency a presumption in the law that attaches to an individual when that person reaches the age of majority. Competence is judged by different standards depending on the context, that is, competence to make a will, to contract, to stand trial, or to make a health-care decision.

decisional capacity the skills, cognitive abilities, and judgment that permit a client, or patient, to address a choice regarding a life situation or care or treatment option.

guardian *ad litem* a special guardian appointed by a court, and considered an officer of the court, whose role it is to represent the interests of an alleged incompetent or adjudicated incompetent during the course of litigation. It is often unclear whether such guardians are to act as advocates of the articulated choices of the alleged or adjudicated incompetent or whether they are to act as more objective, independent fact finders for the court.

References

Dubler, N. N. Fall 1982. The patient's and family's right to know. *Generations*, 1:11–13.

Krauskopf, J. M. 1983. *Advocacy for the aging.* St. Paul, Minn.: West Publishing Co.

Melnick, V. L., and Dubler, N. N., eds. 1985. *Alzheimer's dementia: dilemmas in clinical research.* Clifton, N.J.: Humana Press.

President's Commission for the Study of Ethical Problems in Medicine and Biomedical and Behavioral Research. 1981. *Making Health Care Decisions,* vol. I.

Regan, J. J. 1985. *Tax estate and financial planning for the elderly.* New York: Matthew Bender & Co., Inc.

Schlesinger, S. J. 1984. *Estate planning for the elderly client.* New York: Wiley Law Publications.

CHAPTER EIGHTEEN

Legal Planning for Alzheimer's Disease

Michael Gilfix, J.D.

DEMENTIA IS A CONDITION OF losses: loss of memory, loss of capacities, loss of control, and economic losses. Timely, appropriate, and competent legal advice can make the difference between family destitution and solvency, between respectful decision making by family members and court-imposed decisions, and between appropriate limitations on life-sustaining treatments and the imposition of unwanted medical treatment. Individuals and families can and should plan ahead for the inexorable disability that occurs in the course of Alzheimer's disease (AD) and related dementias, and this chapter will examine the fundamental legal tools and choices that are available to them. Meet with your family legal adviser as soon as possible to decide which of these options you should choose. Early planning is essential. Please

The author gratefully acknowledges the assistance and suggestions provided by Robert Kruger, Esq., and Peter J. Strauss, Esq., both of New York City, in preparation of this chapter.

be aware that laws do vary from state to state, and information in this chapter will have to be interpreted accordingly.

Before examining specific planning options, you must understand the concept of "legal capacity." To be able to sign a will, trust, or power of attorney, a person must understand the nature of the document he is about to sign. He must also understand what it affects and to whom authority is to be given or assets conveyed (by gift or upon death). Significantly, the capacity to understand is not an all-or-nothing phenomenon. Although family members may believe that a patient has lost this capacity, in fact the patient may have significant reserves of understanding. A family's legal adviser will, in many cases, contact the patient's physician and make his or her own determination of capacity. Where capacity is absent, the family may have to rely on the court system.

Legal Tools for Asset Management and Estate Planning

WILLS

A will is the traditional way of planning for distribution of one's assets upon death. *Implemented only upon death* of the individual, the will contains a bequest plan and, possibly, tax-planning options. A will is the traditional estate-planning device; in the natural order of things, people age, get sick, and die, and the estate is distributed by probating the will. A dementing illness is alien to this natural order.

While a will or trust, as discussed below, is preferable for everyone—well, ill, or demented (assuming some mental capacity)—it is absolutely essential for the caregiving spouse, who, in many cases, should be advised that the demented spouse should be given as little as possible. Gifts will only delay eligibility for government entitlements that the demented spouse might need and be eligible for.

DURABLE POWER OF ATTORNEY

A durable power of attorney (DPA) is a legal document that allows a person to choose the person or persons who are to have access to and the legal right to manage his or her personal and business affairs in the event of incapacity. The DPA is a versatile document; it enables the family to manage the property of the incapacitated. It may, for example, include the power to write checks and pay bills, make deposits, and buy and sell securities and other property. In some states, a power of attorney does not empower the attorney to make gifts of property. This is an important distinction; in these states, transfers of assets for Medicaid-eligibility purposes cannot lawfully be made by a person holding a power of attorney.

If properly prepared early in the course of the illness, the DPA can virtually eliminate the need for a guardianship or conservatorship by establishing an alternative method of substitute management. Available in almost every state, it can be signed by any adult who has legal capacity. The DPA also lets the adult exercise personal control by including any restrictions or special instructions in the implementation or use of the document.

Because this document is so important, you should heed two warnings in particular. First, the DPA is private and very powerful. Its power should be given only to a trusted person, as he or she will have no supervision. In the wrong hands, it is a power that can be abused: you might prefer court-supervised conservatorship or guardianship if you know of no capable or trustworthy persons to whom you would give a DPA.

Second, some banks and other financial institutions do not accept blanket DPAs. Whenever a DPA is to be relied upon, its acceptability must be verified with each such institution. Where necessary, other forms, such as stock-and-bond powers, are required to ensure access by the designated substitute person in the event of incapacity. Some states, New York, for example, have recently solved this problem by legislation requiring banks to use and rely on uniform DPA forms. This, however, is not the norm. Verifying acceptability of DPAs is still advisable.

LIVING TRUST

A living trust is a legal planning tool that is created by an individual or couple to ensure the ongoing management of the creator's assets by designated trustees, or trust managers, in the event of the creator's incapacity or death. It also establishes a private bequest plan and method for distribution of assets upon death of the creator(s). The living trust effectively avoids conservatorship while simultaneously avoiding probate.

A living trust includes a bequest plan, as does a will. The critical difference is that a will inevitably involves the costly and sometimes difficult probate process. Trusts are private documents that avoid the court system entirely. Of most importance to families with Alzheimer patients, however, is that a trust enables the families to *conserve* assets and avoid impoverishment.

Such trusts are well established in practice and in the law. For these reasons, a well-drafted trust can be even more effective than a DPA, which is not a conservation tool, in achieving the goals that are important to an Alzheimer family. Since the establishment of a trust may affect eligibility for Medicaid reimbursement, the family would be well advised to seek a counsel knowledgeable about Medicaid and other entitlement programs as well as other, more traditional aspects of estate planning.

STANDBY TRUST

Some families are willing to do financial planning long before the onset of an incapacitating illness. The execution of a standby living trust, a living trust with one difference (compared to the trusts discussed in the preceding paragraphs), may be appropriate.

This trust is created by signing a trust agreement, but it is only nominally funded by transferring as little as $50 or $100 into it at the outset. As the Alzheimer patient gets older, more funds can be transferred into the trust to meet the family's needs as they arise. (Remember, however, a DPA cannot always be used to transfer all family assets into the trust.) Called a "standby trust" because it is ready when needed, this trust can be effective for Medicaid planning purposes and it provides still another way to plan for incapacity without prematurely divesting the family of control.

JOINT BANK ACCOUNTS

Many families, in an attempt to avoid hiring lawyers and to keep things simple, try to ensure access to their bank accounts and other assets by adding their children's names to such accounts. This approach is deceptively attractive and should be undertaken only with great caution. Some of the basic drawbacks are as follows:

1. Anyone named on such an account has complete access to it. A joint account can also be considered an asset of each person; a joint account of an Alzheimer patient and his child may therefore attract creditors who may be owed money by the child.

2. A joint bank account may frustrate the elder's estate plan in that a surviving joint owner typically becomes sole owner of the asset upon death of the elder. A will may have called for equal distribution to all children,

but if only one child's name is on the account, the other children will receive nothing.

3. Depending on the nature of the asset, passing assets along to survivors by this method may strip them of tax benefits that would result if the asset is taken under a will or through a living trust.

4. Most important, in many states a joint account is a "resource" for Medicaid purposes. The entire asset may be forfeited when, not if, expenses increase and Medicaid is applied for.

CONSERVATORSHIP AND GUARDIANSHIP

Conservatorship and guardianship are court-supervised proceedings that determine the Alzheimer patient's limitations in caring for himself or herself or his or her personal finances. The court designates an individual to assume management of the impaired person's affairs and/or personal well-being. These terms are sometimes used interchangeably but do have different meanings in different states. In some states, guardianship may apply only to minors, while conservatorship applies only to adults. In others, guardianship may apply only where personal-care needs of the individual are at issue, while conservatorship pertains to the estate and business matters.

State nuances notwithstanding, both terms apply to court-supervised proceedings where the impaired person is found unable to care for himself or herself or manage his or her personal finances. Hearings must take place to determine such limitations and needs. A psychiatrist is often required. In some states, the impaired person is represented by a court-appointed guardian. The estate pays for everything, and the court examines the patient's actual ability—or inability—to get along in the world. People who are aggrieved by the court's decision can appeal it.

These procedures can serve an appropriate protective function when there is neither a relative nor a trusted friend to assume management of the person's affairs through a power of attorney or a living trust. Conservatorships can also protect the interests of the impaired person from those family members more concerned with their own self-interest than the interest of their relative. However, conservatorships are costly and time-consuming. The DPA, obviously, is preferable in terms of speed.

Some conservatorships or guardianships are unavoidable in many states, where "wandering" Alzheimer patients cannot be placed in locked nursing homes without court authorization. Significantly, in some states the patient can sign a "nomination of conservatorship" document in advance and thereby effectively choose the person who ultimately serves as conservator.

Special Considerations If a Spouse Is in a Nursing Home

Where one spouse is in a nursing home or may soon be, the other spouse should consider whether or not to leave any of his or her estate to the mate. Particularly if the institutionalized spouse is receiving Medicaid coverage for nursing-home bills, a bequest could interfere with Medicaid eligibility and essentially constitute a gift to the nursing home. Thus, the noninstitutionalized spouse may prefer to leave nothing to the other. The mate, however, cannot completely disinherit the spouse in most states. A properly drafted will can accommodate these objectives.

Planning for Public Benefits/Entitlements

The cost of long-term care typically exceeds the ability to pay, and alternative sources of funds are not readily available. Medicare and private insurance pay less than 2 percent of nursing-home bills in America. The balance is paid by care recipients or by the Medicaid program. Medicaid is a federal program administered by the states, and rules vary from state to state. What follows is a discussion of strategies designed to preserve as much of a family's estate as possible while simultaneously qualifying the institutionalized person for Medicaid as quickly as possible.

Some reservations about the entitlements programs must be expressed, however. First, many nursing homes do not accept Medicaid patients at all. Of those that do accept Medicaid, many favor applicants who have funds to pay for a minimum number of months at the private rate. A lack of private funds can therefore severely restrict one's choice of nursing homes.

Second, care must be taken to respect the rights of the Alzheimer patient. While most planning steps are appropriate for most situations and while attention legitimately focuses on the well spouse in addition to the patient, no formulas are automatic or foolproof. You must examine all alternatives and apply them with care on a case-by-case basis.

QUALIFYING FOR MEDICAID

Medicaid is a program based on financial need. To qualify, a person must have sufficiently low levels of income (interest, dividends, social security, pension) and assets (bank accounts, securities, cash surrender value of life insurance, real property other than a home, which is exempt) to be considered "medically indigent." Additionally, the applicant must be a resident of the state, which can be a problem for children whose parents are living in the Sunbelt states when afflicted. For example, Florida has relatively few nursing-home beds. To obtain admission to a nursing home, the parents may wish to move back and obtain a nursing-home bed in the jurisdiction in which they originally resided. Nursing homes may not admit persons who will depend on Medicaid, because of the doubtful residence in the original state, but this is not an insoluble problem. A few months' residence will satisfy the requirements of most nursing homes, but it is not an automatic entry.

In all cases, however, an individual must satisfy the asset requirement, which varies from state to state and is typically in the area of $1,700–$3,000. A couple can possess more assets if both are seeking Medicaid, but it is typically the Alzheimer patient who is in a nursing home and therefore applies for Medicaid *as an individual;* his or her spouse continues to live at home, and neither applies for nor qualifies for Medicaid. The significance of this fact becomes clear with the division of assets.

A person can have income over the monthly income limit and still receive Medicaid in some states if the monthly medical and nursing-home bills exceed his or her ability to pay. This applies in New York, for example. In such cases, the person typically pays his or her income to the nursing home, and the Medicaid program pays the balance. This is the typical situation for Alzheimer patients who have some income but not enough to pay all nursing-home bills. States such as New Jersey and Florida, on the other hand, have a different rule: if the patient's income exceeds eligibility limits, the patient is disqualified, without recourse.

EXEMPT ASSETS

How do you determine your assets? Not all assets are counted in determining eligibility. The home is typically exempt, irrespective of value, so long as the Medicaid applicant or his or her spouse or dependent or disabled children actually live in it or will soon return to it. The home may be exempt—an applicant can be eligible for Medicaid if he or she owns a home—but it is not immune. On death, the state can file a claim against the estate as a creditor, and the state will collect on its claim. Other exempt assets include modest life insurance, a burial trust fund, a burial plot, and the family car.

One possible approach for improving eligibility potential is to convert a nonexempt asset, such as cash, to an exempt form. If a couple does not own a home, for example, their exempt cash can be used to purchase one. If they already own a home, it may be wise to improve it. In this way, funds can be put into a "safe harbor" even while the Alzheimer patient is applying for Medicaid.

SPENDING DOWN

So long as fair value is received, assets can be spent and thereby reduced until they meet eligibility requirements. This is important for persons who have relatively few disqualifying assets. Thus, furniture can be purchased, or appliances, but gifts cannot be given to achieve instant eligibility.

GIFTS

So long as the patient has capacity, gifting can preserve assets if the "two-year rule" is respected. In most states, Medicaid only inquires into gifts that were made in the two-year period preceding the date of application. If a gift was made within two years of applying for Medicaid, eligibility will be denied. Gifts made more than two years before application usually pose far fewer problems.

What factors must a patient consider before making gifts? First, understand that a gift is a complete, irreversible, "no strings attached" transfer of money or other assets. While a mother with AD may transfer her assets to her children as gifts and feel confident that they will reciprocate by giving her money if she needs it, she must understand that they are not legally required to do so.

Another consideration is possible stress on the family. When the well spouse, in particular, needs the unfettered love and support of her family, might gifts from the spouse with AD interfere with an existing supportive relationship? Money can cause stress, worry, and concern if not handled wisely. If a husband with AD makes a gift to a child with a "spendthrift" history, for example, it may cause his wife more worry than if she kept the money, divided it, and spent half on her husband's care.

No less important is the well spouse's feeling of independence, which can be threatened if she no longer holds her assets because her husband has gifted them. Rightly or wrongly, in our society money is often equated with control of one's life. This social or psychological factor can generate potentially significant worries.

Gifting to preserve assets may, in other words, be a necessary and effective strategy to preserve one's assets, but it must not be undertaken without considering the human factors that are involved.

DIVISION OF ASSETS

Under Medicaid rules in many states, half of the family assets (other than the home) can usually be preserved where the patient has a living spouse. To achieve this, the well spouse divides the assets with the institutionalized spouse. The well spouse keeps his or her half, and the patient is put on Medicaid after exhausting his or her resources.

Some states, such as California, allow an "automatic" division of such assets when one spouse enters a nursing home. Court approval of a division may be needed in some states to take maximum advantage of this benefit. Therefore, dividing the assets beforehand is clearly preferable.

Limiting Estate or Inheritance Taxes

As of 1987, each individual can leave an estate worth up to $600,000 without any federal "death taxes." An unlimited amount can be left to a surviving spouse. With proper planning, a family estate of up to $1.2 million can be left to children and other heirs without any federal taxes whatsoever. State inheritance and estate taxes vary widely and must be independently reviewed.

While not a planning concern of most families who now face no such taxes, it is a source of inappropriate cases. Use of a "bypass" trust, which can be in a will or a living trust, achieves maximum ($1.2 million) protection.

When an estate exceeds this figure, *gifting* should be considered to reduce the estate to a nontaxable level. A couple can annually give away up to $20,000 per recipient ($10,000 each) without incurring any federal gift taxes. State laws vary.

DIVORCE OR LEGAL SEPARATION

Although still advised by many lawyers, divorce or legal separation is almost never necessary as a strategy to preserve one's assets. In some cases, this personally and legally radical step can even expose the family to economic risk.

You should note first that many assets can be preserved without divorce. Who owns the property, that is, who has title, is of primary importance. A court-supervised separation does result in division of assets and could compel sale and division of the family home. Medicaid rules treat the residence as an exempt asset and preserve it for the well spouse as long as he or she is alive.

Moreover, in a divorce, a judge could order the well spouse to pay spousal support for the Alzheimer patient in a long-term-care facility. Medicaid income rules also mandate contributions for support by the well spouse but may, in certain cases, be more protective of the well spouse.

No less significant is the potential emotional hurt that can result from dissolution of a long-term marriage. No matter what the economic circumstances are, this vulnerability is a vital consideration.

TRANSFER OF THE RESIDENCE

The residence is an exempt asset. Nevertheless, transfer out of the Alzheimer patient's name and into the name of the spouse can have salutary effects without harming the patient. This can be done without imposition of the two-year "no transfer" rule and can therefore be accomplished at any time. However, it should be done prior to institutionalization and before the patient receives Medicaid benefits.

If the home is in the well spouse's name, he or she can sell the residence and keep all proceeds, because Medicaid rules do not include his or her *separate* property in determining the spouse's eligibility. If the home were held in both names and sold, half of the proceeds (now nonexempt cash) would go to the patient and thereby end Medicaid eligibility.

If the residence is in the well spouse's name, additional transfer may be required to protect the home from state efforts to recapture Medicaid benefits upon the death of the spouse. Although the assets would not be in the recipient's name, some states have filed claims against the estate of the spouse, and a few have enforced their claims.

Emerging Issues

LONG-TERM-CARE INSURANCE

Reimbursement for long-term-care services is not widely available, with very limited coverage under Medicare, and Medicaid providing coverage only for those who are eligible. Private coverage plans are beginning to emerge. The sketchy information presently available suggests that such insurance is no panacea. For example, per diem payments are nowhere near the $110–$150 per diem costs in the Northeast; most plans exclude coverage for preexisting conditions; some plans have unrealistically low maximum benefits or time limitations. The extent of coverage and benefits varies radically. No policy should be purchased without a careful and complete comparison of all policies that exist.

LEGAL TOOLS FOR HEALTH-CARE DECISION MAKING

Everyone is concerned about how they will be treated in the event of terminal illness, coma, or hopeless dementia. The absence of decision-making ability in such circumstances presents the issue even more starkly as more and more older Americans are kept alive through the wonder of "high tech" medicine and improvements in chronic-care procedures. The Alzheimer patient will eventually become unable to make day-to-day health-care decisions as well as those relating to "life-sustaining" procedures. Some patients may be able to plan for this eventuality by signing appropriate documents in advance of incapacity. With earlier diagnoses, this practice will become more widespread.

LIVING WILLS

A "living will" is a generic term that describes a document in which a patient indicates that life-sustaining treatments are not to be used in certain circumstances. The best form of a living will varies from state to state, as some states have specific laws authorizing them, while others do not. Requirements and prerequisites also vary in different jurisdictions.

Such documents can be useful only if their existence is

known, and copies should be distributed to all medical-care providers. Types of life-sustaining treatment that might be addressed include: nasogastric tube feeding, use of respirator, dialysis, antibiotics, and resuscitation. In no event, however, should a living will be relied upon to the exclusion of *discussion* with attending physicians about the course of medical treatment. Individual physicians' attitudes about living wills vary tremendously and must be understood. If, for example, a physician is disinclined to honor a patient's lawful wishes—whatever they may be—transfer to a different physician may be necessary.

The living will is available throughout the United States, but should not be used where state law provides for a more reliable or legally enforceable document such as the DPAHC.

DURABLE POWERS OF ATTORNEY FOR HEALTH CARE (DPAHC)

Only available in some jurisdictions, DPAHCs represent an excellent vehicle for surrogate health-care decision making. In this document, an individual chooses the person(s) who will make health-care decisions for him or her in the event of incapacity and may also explain how decisions are to be made. This instruction can specifically address use or nonuse of life-sustaining treatment.

Some uses of the DPAHC include authorization for access to medical records, disclosure of medical information, and the authority to employ and discharge medical personnel, consent to specific procedures, arrange for care in a nursing home, hospital, or hospice, authorize or refuse life-sustaining equipment, withdraw life-support systems, and medicate to relieve pain. Since future needs are unpredictable and the issues of the moment often cannot be programmed in advance, a DPAHC gives far greater flexibility than a living will, which usually deals with life-support systems and use of heroic measures to sustain life and little more.

The Lawyer as a Member of the Health-Care Team

Only by taking full and aggressive advantage of legal planning options can the losses associated with AD be minimized and control restored to the family. Certain steps—the DPA, a living will, DPAHC, or Medicaid planning—should be taken by everyone presented with an Alzheimer problem. Other options, such as the living trust and a decision about which Medicaid options to pursue, depend on individual circumstances.

Being aware of the myriad issues confronting the family is the first step toward resolving them. This chapter has identified them and can serve as something of a checklist for families seeking legal assistance. Above all, families must be informed, they must act, and they must assume responsibility. Otherwise, events and circumstances can become overwhelming and only add to the losses that already threaten to take control of their lives.

Glossary

durable power of attorney a legal document that allows a person to choose the person or persons who are to have access to, and the legal right to manage, personal and business affairs in the event of incapacity.

durable power of attorney for health care similar to the durable power of attorney. This document lets an individual choose a person who will have the power to make health-care decisions in the event of incapacity.

living trust a legal planning tool created by an individual or couple to ensure the ongoing management and conservation of the individual's or couple's assets by designated persons (trustees) in the event of the creator's incapacity or death. The trust also may avoid the probate process by establishing a private bequest plan and method for distribution of assets upon death of the creator(s).

conservatorship and guardianship court-supervised proceedings that determine one's limitations in caring for himself or herself or his or her personal finances. The court designates an individual to assume management of the impaired person's affairs and/or personal well-being.

CHAPTER NINETEEN

Government-Funded Programs to Finance Care for Patients and Families

David F. Chavkin, J.D.

THE ONSET OF ALZHEIMER'S disease (AD) or a related disorder creates enormous pressures for the family involved. These pressures could be lessened somewhat if the financing and delivery system for needed care and services adequately addressed family needs. Unfortunately, this system often increases the problems confronting those affected. However, valuable and available assistance *can* be obtained through positive action and perseverance on the part of the family.

This chapter reviews the current entitlement programs available to finance some of the needed care and services for persons with (AD) and their families. It will also highlight some of the special problems facing persons with dementia and suggest some approaches that can be used to address these problems.

When evaluating any of the entitlement programs, you must first ask four types of questions:

293

1. Who is eligible under the program? What special eligibility criteria does an applicant have to satisfy?
2. What do recipients receive as benefits? Do they receive cash payments, direct services, or reimbursement to third parties for services?
3. What agencies dispense benefits to recipients? Is the program administered by the federal government, the state, the county, or some other agency?
4. What must recipients do to continue to receive those benefits? What are the requirements for continuing eligibility under the program?

Financial Entitlements

When a family member experiences the onset of dementia, one of the first problems the family may have to address is the need for additional financial support. If it is the wage earner who is affected by AD or a related disorder, the lost wages will need to be replaced. If the spouse who maintains the home and raises the children is affected, financial support will be needed to pay someone to perform that spouse's tasks.

There are four major financial entitlement programs available to meet some of these needs. Keep in mind that the distinguishing feature of an entitlement program is that all persons who meet eligibility criteria must be determined eligible for services. Two of these programs, Social Security benefits and Supplemental Security Income, are administered by the Social Security Administration. The other two programs, Aid to Families with Dependent Children (AFDC) and General Public Assistance, are administered by the various states and localities.

SOCIAL SECURITY BENEFITS

The Social Security Administration administers a variety of social insurance programs. The distinguishing feature of a social insurance program is that there are no limits on the amount of other income or resources that an applicant may have to be eligible. In social welfare jargon, there is no "means test" for Social Security eligibility. There are, however, other strict eligibility requirements.

The Social Security social insurance programs are all reflected in the initials OASDHI. As with many federal and state programs, applicants and recipients who can master the "alphabet soup" of these programs will generally be in the best shape in establishing and maintaining eligibility.

The OA part of *OAS*DHI stands for old-age benefits. These are benefits for wage earners who are at least sixty-two years of age. Since age is usually an easy factor to demonstrate, Social Security eligibility for a person with dementia who is at least sixty-two usually presents no problems.

The S part of OAS*D*HI stands for survivor's benefits. These are benefits paid to the spouse and/or children of deceased workers and are calculated based on the Social Security taxes paid by the wage earner when working. The HI part of OASD*HI* stands for health insurance, known popularly as Medicare. This program of medical insurance is discussed later in the chapter.

SOCIAL SECURITY DISABILITY

The D part of OASD*H*I stands for disability benefits. Social Security disability (SSDI) is a social insurance program designed to protect wage earners who can no longer engage in substantial gainful employment. This is the major program available to wage earners disabled by dementia who are under age sixty-two.

The first major requirement for SSDI is that an applicant must have worked a sufficient number of covered quarters before becoming disabled. In general, an applicant must have worked at least twenty quarters during the forty-quarter period ending with the quarter in which the disability began. These quarters need not have been worked consecutively.

However, if an applicant waits too long to apply for disability benefits after becoming disabled, this "twenty/forty" work requirement may no longer be met.

The second major requirement is that the applicant must be prevented from engaging in substantial gainful activity by reason of a "medically determinable physical or mental impairment that can be expected to last for a continuous period of not less than twelve months." This definition presents special problems for applicants suffering from AD.

One of the major problems with AD is the present inability to diagnose the disease positively while the applicant is still alive. It may, therefore, be impossible for the applicant to demonstrate that the impairment is "medically determinable."

These problems are compounded because AD is not yet included in the "Listing of Impairments." The listing describes impairments that are severe enough to preclude an individual from engaging in substantial gainful activity, yet Alzheimer applicants must individually demonstrate that they are functionally disabled.

Another problem for applicants is the waiting period for benefits. Under federal law, a waiting period of five consecutive months after the onset of the illness is imposed before benefits can be initiated. An applicant will therefore have to rely on other sources of income for at least this five-month period.

The potential delays are far greater, however. Many applicants for Social Security disability benefits are turned down on initial application. Unless these applicants pursue their appeal rights by filing a request for reconsideration, a request for a hearing before an administrative law judge if reconsideration is denied, a request for Appeals Council review if the hearing is denied, and a petition for judicial review if the Appeals Council review is unfavorable, benefits may never be granted.

A reconsideration is a paper review by an individual not

directly involved in the prior denial. Applicants can submit additional medical documentation at this stage. The hearing stage provides an opportunity for review by an independent hearing officer. Oral and written testimony can be presented. The applicant can be assisted by family members and friends and by an attorney or paralegal. The last two stages, Appeals Council and judicial review, provide more limited opportunities for applicants to demonstrate that denial was improper.

These various stages of review are critical if eligibility is to be established. For example, approximately 50 percent of all denials are overturned at the administrative hearing stage. However, fewer than 10 percent of denials are appealed. It is therefore crucial for a family to persevere in seeking Social Security benefits and not to give up early in the process.

Once eligibility is established, an applicant receives a payment each month based on his or her earnings record. In general, these benefits are far greater than those under any of the comparable social welfare programs.

SUPPLEMENTAL SECURITY INCOME

In addition to the social insurance programs outlined above, the Social Security Administration also administers a social welfare program called Supplemental Security Income (SSI). The SSI program provides a minimum federal benefit level nationwide of $340 per month in 1987, generally adjusted annually for inflation. In addition, some states supplement the federal benefit for certain classes of recipients.

Persons with dementia who are dependent on SSI benefits are generally those who have no recent work history (making them ineligible for Social Security disability benefits) or who were employed in low-paying jobs (making them eligible for only a small Social Security disability benefit). For this latter class of recipients, SSI benefits can be used to supplement SSDI benefits.

Applicants for SSI benefits face all of the difficulties encountered by applicants for SSDI benefits, with additional problems, as well. SSI applicants must meet all of the same disability criteria as applicants for SSDI benefits. However, because SSI is a social welfare program, SSI applicants must meet all of the "means test" criteria imposed under the program.

For example, an SSI recipient must own less than $1,800 in liquid assets such as a bank account or stocks and bonds, plus a $1,500 separately titled and segregated burial fund. This requirement alone will immediately exclude most middle-class families from eligibility, or at least until they have impoverished themselves by spending nearly all of their assets for needed care and services.

Once they are eligible, the picture is not much brighter. In most states, an SSI recipient will receive only $340 per month in the community. Any outside income received by the recipient, after a small income disregard, will be used to reduce the SSI payment. This means that the recipient will be forced to live far below the poverty level even after being certified for assistance.

AID TO FAMILIES WITH DEPENDENT CHILDREN (AFDC)

Although most persons affected by AD and related disorders are over the age of sixty, many persons are affected in their forties and fifties. For those younger persons with children under the age of eighteen, AFDC may be the only financial support available.

AFDC is a social welfare program for children deprived of parental support by reason of the death, physical or mental incapacity, continued absence, or, in many states, unemployment of a parent. Payments also cover the caretaker relatives with whom the children are living. AFDC is governed by both federal and state regulations.

Those persons with dementia who are unable to meet the Social Security disability criteria can usually still meet the easier AFDC "mental incapacity" requirements. However, the other eligibility requirements are stringent. The definition of "mental incapacity" may differ from state to state.

A family of six on AFDC can own less than half as much in liquid assets as a couple on SSI. Similarly, the AFDC grant levels for a family of three in about half the states are less than the SSI grant level for an individual. For families with no alternative, however, AFDC benefits may represent the best and only source of financial assistance.

GENERAL PUBLIC ASSISTANCE

The SSI and AFDC programs are social welfare programs that depend to a large extent on federal financial assistance. Nearly all of the costs of the SSI program are paid for by the federal government, while between one-half and three-quarters of the costs of the AFDC program are federally funded.

Unfortunately, not all needy persons are eligible for SSI or AFDC. A person with dementia under sixty-five who cannot meet Social Security disability criteria and who does not have a child at home is ineligible for both SSI and AFDC. This individual may therefore be dependent on General Public Assistance.

General Public Assistance is a social welfare program for indigent persons financed solely by state and/or local funds. It is known by different names in different jurisdictions. It may be called general relief or home relief, but regardless of its name, it is a program of assistance for those indigent persons who cannot qualify for any other welfare program.

As restrictive as requirements under the SSI and AFDC programs may be, they appear generous when compared with those under General Public Assistance. Benefits under this program are frequently less than one hundred dollars per month and may be limited to only three months' duration. For those persons with no other choice, however, General Public Assistance may be the last source of any financial support. It is also commonly used as the interim funding source while Social Security and SSI applicants are being processed.

Entitlements

Just as there are social insurance and social welfare programs providing financial support, there are social insurance and social welfare programs providing assistance with medical costs. The two major programs are the Medicare and Medicaid programs.

MEDICARE

The Medicare program is a social insurance program administered by the Health Care Financing Administration (HCFA) of the U.S. Department of Health and Human Services through a network of fiscal intermediaries and carriers. Eligibility for the Medicare program "piggybacks" on the Social Security social insurance programs.

In order to be eligible for Medicare, an individual must be a recipient of Social Security old-age benefits (i.e., he or she must be over the age of sixty-five) or must have been a recipient of Social Security disability benefits for at least twenty-four months. This means that an individual with dementia under the age of sixty-five will not be able to receive Medicare benefits until nearly 2½ years (a five-month waiting period for Social Security disability benefits plus a twenty-four-month waiting period while on the Social Security disability program) after the disability has become severe enough to prevent gainful employment.

Once eligible for Medicare, a beneficiary is eligible for

benefits under Parts A and B. Part A is without charge to the insured. There is a fee for Part B. The major benefit under Part A is reimbursement for inpatient hospital care. The Medicare program will cover up to ninety days of medically necessary inpatient hospital care in each benefit period plus a lifetime reserve of sixty hospital days. This means that Medicare will provide reimbursement for up to 150 days of coverage in a single hospital stay. This coverage is not without limitations, however. The 1987 premium is $17.90 per month.

The beneficiary remains liable for the average cost of the first day of hospitalization, $520 in 1987, during the first sixty days of hospitalization. This is the inpatient deductible. During the next thirty days, the beneficiary must pay a cost of $130 per day, as of 1987. Finally, during the reserve days, if any, the beneficiary must pay another cost, $260 per day, as of 1987. A lengthy hospital stay may therefore mean significant costs for the beneficiary unless other insurance is available.

The major benefit under Part B is reimbursement for physician's services. The Medicare program will pay for 80 percent of the approved fee for a physician. The beneficiary is liable for the remainder. This means that if a physician's actual charge is forty dollars for a visit and the approved fee is thirty dollars, the maximum Medicare reimbursement is twenty-four dollars (80 percent of thirty dollars). The beneficiary would then be liable for the remaining sixteen dollars ($40 − $24).

The only exception to this stipulation is if the physician agrees to accept assignment. The relatively small percentage of physicians who accept assignment agree to accept the Medicare-approved fee as payment in full. In such cases the beneficiary is obligated to pay only the remaining 20 percent of the approved fee, or six dollars in the previous example. Some areas have directories of those physicians who accept assignment, but these are few and far between.

The major benefit not covered by either Part A or B is nursing-home care. Although the Medicare program does cover some skilled nursing-facility care, most nursing-home care for patients with dementia is not covered. Requests for reimbursement are generally denied on the basis that the care required by a patient with AD is "custodial" in nature, as opposed to skilled nursing care.

Medicare beneficiaries have appeal rights similar to those of other Social Security beneficiaries. When applicants challenge the denied-coverage dictum, many beneficiaries receive coverage for at least a portion of their stay, since such services as skilled observation and administration of medications on an as-needed basis are considered skilled nursing services. Here again, applicants' perseverance is crucial.

Even perseverance, however, cannot alter the fact that many of the services needed by a person with dementia are simply not covered under the Medicare program. This is especially true for the younger person with dementia who must undergo a 2½-year wait before establishing Medicare eligibility. By the time that waiting period has been exhausted, all of the needed diagnostic and assessment services have probably been provided. What are really needed then are personal-care services, respite services, day-care services, and intermediate nursing care. None of these services are covered under Medicare.

MEDICAID

The Medicaid program is a social welfare program administered by the states with federal financial assistance. Both the types of persons eligible for benefits and the benefits covered vary widely from state to state within minimum federal requirements.

Just as Medicare eligibility "piggybacks" on Social Security old-age and disability eligibility, so does Medicaid eligibility "piggyback" on SSI and AFDC eligibility. This means that in most states all recipients of SSI and AFDC benefits automatically get Medicaid benefits as well.

In addition to recipients of cash welfare benefits, most states also provide optional Medicaid eligibility to persons with high medical expenses whose income and/or resources disqualify them from cash welfare. In some states, eligibility is limited to those persons in nursing homes with incomes less than three times the SSI benefit level. In other states, eligibility is available in the community or in institutions for those persons whose high medical expenses reduce their available incomes below a specified level. This latter class of persons is known as the medically needy.

Establishing financial eligibility is a major problem for many persons with dementia. Although excess income can be reduced by incurring sufficient medical expenses, there is no comparable spend-down for resources. Since Medicaid resource limits generally parallel the cash welfare program limits, any substantial savings will have to be eliminated before eligibility can be established.

Similar problems arise with income eligibility. Ordinarily, the eligibility of an applicant living in the community will be determined in light of the income and resources of all related persons with whom the applicant is living. To the extent that these persons have any income and resources of their own, eligibility for the applicant with dementia will usually not be possible.

A different situation is presented if the applicant is institutionalized. Beginning with the first day of the first full month of institutionalization, in most states, the applicant's eligibility will be determined solely on the basis of his or her income and resources. Income of a noninstitutionalized spouse is no longer "deemed" or presumed available to the institutionalized spouse. This is one of the reasons why the Medicaid program is often criticized as having a bias toward institutionalization.

Although the Medicaid program encourages institutionalization if the noninstitutionalized spouse has income, real hardship is created if the income is in the name of the institutionalized spouse. In most states, the noninstitutionalized spouse will be permitted to receive only $340 (the SSI benefit level) from the institutionalized spouse's income. Any income received by the noninstitutionalized spouse would reduce this allocation. As a result, impoverishment of the noninstitutionalized spouse is ensured in many cases.

Once an applicant is deemed eligible, he or she may find that the scope of Medicaid-covered services may pose further problems. Although all states provide a range of institutional and noninstitutional services, many states do not cover respite care, personal care, or adult day health care. Other states impose limits on the amount, duration, and scope of services, which may create additional difficulties. Services such as physician care may be limited to one visit per month. In such states, these limits may greatly diminish the value of Medicaid coverage for a person with dementia.

Even the coverage of a service under the state plan does not guarantee reimbursement. Many providers are unwilling to accept Medicaid patients. Access to providers of covered services is especially difficult for certain classes of recipients, especially minority persons. If you are denied access, you have appeal rights guaranteed by state and federal laws.

Other Programs

The distinguishing feature of an "entitlement" program is that all persons who meet eligibility criteria must be determined eligible for services. Although such "entitlement" programs as SSI and Medicaid are important for persons with dementia and other elderly and disabled individuals, families should not lose sight of the "discretionary" programs that can help provide assistance.

The two major discretionary programs affecting persons with dementia are the Older Americans Act and the Social Services Block Grant. Each of these federal programs provides financial assistance to those states that submit approved plans. All states now have such plans.

Although these two programs have slightly different target populations, there is also significant overlap. The Older Americans Act is targeted at those persons sixty years of age and older. The Social Services Block Grant is targeted at low-income children and adults. Both programs, therefore, provide assistance to low-income elderly persons.

In most states, the Older Americans Act funding is provided through Area Agencies on Aging. By contrast, the Social Services Block Grant funding is generally provided through local departments of social services. Generally, both programs have some eligibility process administered by the designated agency.

These programs are important for recipients of entitlement programs and for persons ineligible for those programs. In many states, the discretionary grant programs are utilized to fill in gaps for entitlement recipients. For example, needed services that are not available through the entitlement programs, such as respite care, may be funded through the discretionary grant program. For other persons, the discretionary grants may help purchase services, such as home modifications, that can avoid institutionalization and ultimately reduce the financial burden on the states and federal government.

Lessons for Families

The primary lesson for families is that they should begin thinking about financial eligibility for entitlement and other programs as soon as the symptoms of AD or a related disorder appear. This is critical because financial eligibility for care and services is one of the elements that should be considered as part of a coherent estate plan. Moreover, in many cases the sooner a plan is implemented, the better able family caregivers will be to cope with the needs of the disabled family member.

For example, as discussed in chapter 18, most states require all transfers of assets for less than market value to be made at least two years in advance of applying for assistance. In order to ensure that a healthy spouse is not forced onto the welfare rolls by the institutionalization of the spouse with AD, a coherent estate plan would ensure that sufficient assets are available in the name of the noninstitutionalized spouse to permit a standard of living above the poverty level.

The need to plan with entitlement eligibility in mind is especially important since other financial protection devices are not available. For example, private health insurance can meet many of the costs of health care for most persons. Unfortunately, most of the needs of persons with AD or a related disorder are not covered by private health-insurance policies. Moreover, such alternatives as private long-term-care insurance are too expensive for all but the wealthiest families and provide coverage that is too limited for all but the shortest-term patients.

The second major lesson is the importance of individual perseverance. Unfortunately, the stamina required may already be beyond the capability of a family attempting to cope with a disabled family member. However, the eventual rewards for perseverance are significant. Many applicants for benefits are turned down initially. One recent study found that fewer than 5 percent of the people wrongfully denied benefits ever challenged that denial. Therefore, a strong incentive exists for the Social Security Administration and welfare agencies to initially deny benefits. For those persons who successfully appeal the denial, the agency is only paying money that it was required to pay under the law.

There are many resources available to assist families in

pursuing such claims, thereby taking some of the pressure off the families involved. The Older Americans Act funds legal-services programs for the elderly. The Legal Services Corporation Act funds legal-services programs for indigent persons. In some areas, private attorneys are willing to provide reduced-fee services. Legal clinics or law-school-affiliated programs may also be available. The potential benefits are great if you pursue these legal entitlements with the best resources available.

Glossary

entitlement a program that provides financial or other assistance to all persons who meet program eligibility requirements.

General Public Assistance a social welfare program administered by the states or by localities without federal funding to provide financial assistance to indigents who have no other source of support.

Medicaid a social welfare program administered by the states with partial federal funding that provides reimbursement for certain medical costs incurred by recipients. Medicaid may provide funds for long-term care.

Medicare a social insurance program administered by the Health Care Financing Administration of the U.S. Department of Health and Human Services that provides reimbursement for certain medical costs incurred by beneficiaries. Medicare does not usually provide funds for long-term-care services.

Social Security disability a social insurance program administered by the Social Security Administration of the U.S. Department of Health and Human Services that provides financial assistance to wage earners who can no longer work due to a physical or mental impairment.

Supplemental Security Income a social welfare program administered by the Social Security Administration of the U.S. Department of Health and Human Services that provides financial assistance to indigent persons who are over the age of sixty-five, blind, or totally and permanently disabled.

CHAPTER TWENTY

Rights of
and Duties to
the Terminally Ill

Charles C. Bell, J.D.

RECENT ADVANCES IN THE delivery of health-care services have allowed patients suffering from incurable and irreparable disease to live longer. These same factors also prolong the process of dying. The most poignant personification of these advancements is those patients who linger indefinitely in a permanent vegetative coma. As a result, profound questions of rights and duties to the terminally ill are challenging the medical and legal professions, religious and secular philosophers, health-care planners and providers, and the general public, and there is no unanimity of opinion. Beginning with the Karen Ann Quinlan case in 1974, principles of law have emerged concerning the rights of, and responsibilities to, those afflicted with terminal and irreparable disease. These profound questions are of great significance to the families of persons with Alzheimer's disease (AD) and related disorders.

Informed Consent and the Right to Die

An understanding of these issues begins with the doctrine of informed consent, a fundamental legal principle governing the patient-physician relationship. Before a physician can render treatment to a patient, he or she must obtain the patient's consent. To obtain this consent, the patient must be informed of the nature of the treatment, its risks, its potential benefits, and the risk to the patient if the treatment is refused. A competent patient ordinarily has the right to accept or refuse the recommended treatment. For a patient who is incompetent, suffering from either a temporary or permanent impairment of mental abilities or loss of consciousness, consent to medical treatment is rendered by his legal representative or by his next of kin, or his consent is presumed if emergency medical treatment is required. Refusal of consent to the introduction or continuation of life-sustaining treatment is popularly known as the patient's "right to die."

Termination of Life

The right to die is distinguished from three other forms of termination of life: euthanasia, homicide, and suicide. Euthanasia is defined as taking the life of another to relieve incurable or insufferable pain, performed with a merciful motive. Euthanasia may be "passive," the consequence of withholding medical treatment, with death resulting thereafter, or it may be "active," the consequence of performing an overt act to cause death. The law has neither explicitly condemned nor condoned passive euthanasia, as such, but active euthanasia has been considered an act of homicide. The courts are now grappling with the complex moral and legal issues presented by withholding treatment.

Homicide is the killing of a human being without justification or excuse. A humanitarian motive, or mercy killing, does not justify or excuse an act of homicide.

Suicide, the voluntary taking of one's own life, was historically classified as a criminal act. While suicide is no longer regarded as a crime, aiding or abetting a suicide is generally considered to be a crime in the United States.

Medical Feasibility Versus Futility

The patient's right to die is affected by the physician's duty to render treatment. Once the physician-patient relationship is established and until the physician is discharged by the patient, the physician must exercise reasonable care and good medical practice. Historically, this has meant that the physician had the affirmative responsibility to preserve life and render life-sustaining treatment. In recent times, however, physicians have considered the medical feasibility or medical futility of treatment. This is a "quality of life" issue, which is the medical corollary of the legal "right to die." Medical feasibility is the consideration of the risk of harm to the patient from the administration of medical treatment when weighed against the potential benefit to the patient. Medical futility is defined as the administration of treatment that affords no benefit other than to prolong the act of dying.

The emerging view of the medical profession appears to be that when a patient has a terminal and irreparable condition and death is imminent, anything more than nourishment and relief of pain is considered extraordinary care. However, even with family consent to withhold or remove life-sustaining treatments from incompetent persons, hospitals and physicians have turned to the courts for approval. The courts have had to determine the competency of the patient, whether the patient has expressed his or her views regarding the medical issues presented, who may act on behalf of an incompetent patient, the medical issues involved, whether the court should be involved in questions such as these, and the legal principles under which the controversy is to be decided.

The Right to Refuse Life-Sustaining Treatment

Historically, the state had an absolute interest in maintaining or preserving life, as exemplified by the existing laws prohibiting homicide and aiding or abetting a suicide, and the former laws that punished those who attempted suicide and caused the forfeiture of the estates of those individuals who successfully committed suicide. However, there has been an expansion of the individual's right to self-determination through constitutional protections and broader judicial interpretations of the scope of personal rights, particularly the right to privacy. At the same time, the law recognizes the ramifications of the great improvements in medical care of the chronically ill and the shifting societal attitudes as to what constitutes "life," prolongation of life, and "extraordinary care." Therefore, courts have undertaken careful consideration of the factual circumstances and principles of law concerning the right, in general, to refuse medical treatment and, specifically, the right to refuse life-sustaining treatment.

Presumably, a competent person has the right to refuse life-sustaining treatment. However, in determining whether a competent individual may be treated against his will, courts have considered several factors, including the reasons for his refusal, the impact on his family if treatment is not rendered, the risk of harm to the patient from the treatment, the medical consequences to the patient if treatment is withheld, and the patient's prognosis if the treatment is successful. These same factors are relevant in cases concerning incompetent patients, with the crucial distinction that an incompetent patient cannot express his present wish. In addition, courts have had to determine whether the incompetent patient has expressed any wishes on the subject, who may act on behalf of an incompetent patient, and the scope of authority of the representative to act on behalf of the patient.

Making Medical Decisions for Incompetent Persons

Formally, a guardian or conservator is appointed by the court to make medical decisions for an incompetent person. Presently in many states, it appears that an attorney-in-fact (a person appointed by another to act on his or her behalf) has similar authority under a durable medical power of attorney executed by the patient when competent. The legal representative's authority has traditionally been limited to making medical decisions to improve, sustain, or continue the life of the incompetent. Informally, the patient's next of kin have made decisions to terminate or withhold life-sustaining treatment whenever they have been consulted, thereby avoiding the necessity of court intervention. However, if the hospitals or physicians do not prove accommodating or if family members disagree among themselves, court intervention will occur.

Court Involvement

Courts have ascertained the incompetent's right to refuse life-sustaining treatment under different legal principles. The determinations vary from state to state. For example, New Jersey has determined that the decision is one to be made by the physician and the family. Depending on the circumstances, the hospital may be required to appoint a panel of physicians to review each case. For example, the panel may determine that the patient is in a permanent vegetative state, thereby removing the decision from the physician-patient or physician-family arena. The evolution of the judicial decision is decidedly in favor of removing life-sustaining equipment if the panel has determined that the patient is in a permanent vegetative state.

Massachusetts, while recognizing the patient's right to privacy, requires judicial review of the decision to withhold or remove life-sustaining treatment in order to balance the individual's asserted "right to die" against the interest of the state to preserve life under the specific facts presented. New York has based its decisions on the principle of substituted judgment. Life-sustaining procedures can be withheld or removed only if the patient, when competent, had explicitly expressed such a desire. The state of Washington requires the appointment of a guardian but allows him or her to refuse consent to the administration of life-sustaining treatment for the ward if this would be in the incompetent's "best interest." The "best interest" is the legal standard that governs all decisions of a guardian for the ward.

It should be emphasized that the courts have generally recognized the incompetent's "right to die" only in the limited circumstances when the patient suffers from an irreversible and irreparable illness and death is imminent if life-sustaining treatment, or extraordinary care, is withheld or removed. Following the opinions in the leading cases of *In Re Quinlan* and *In Re Spring*, courts across the country have generally ruled that life-sustaining medical treatment may be terminated if the treatment is futile and the next of kin agree with the doctor to remove or withhold treatment, especially when it is in accord with the expressed desire of the patient when competent.

Legislation

In response to these court decisions, many states have enacted legislation allowing a competent adult to express in writing his intent not to receive extraordinary care if he should become incompetent. This written expression, popularly known as a "living will" (see chapter 18), is generally limited to circumstances of terminal and irreparable illness, when death is imminent and applying life-sustaining procedures would serve only to prolong artificially the process of dying. Individuals who want to execute a living will or durable medical power of attorney should do so while they are competent to express their intent.

Legislative enactments of the living will and the durable medical power of attorney, which is a document of broader authority, would obviate many of the presently existing legal issues in this difficult area.

Table 20.1 shows a living will from the Commonwealth of Virginia, which is a representative sample.

Emerging Definitions

Still, the emerging definitions and limits of the "right to die" continue to raise additional questions. A prominent issue concerns the definition of "extraordinary care." Until recently, this has meant the administration of respirators, dialysis machines, or resuscitative intervention for cardiac arrests. However, the American Medical Association and litigants in New Jersey and Massachusetts have now raised the question as to whether the definition of extraordinary care should be expanded to include food and water for those patients existing in a persistent vegetative coma, even if death is not imminent. Thus, even nutritional treatment is now determined to be medically futile. While it is possible that this policy statement may make withholding all forms of life-sustaining treatment more socially acceptable, the ultimate impact on courts and lawmakers cannot be accurately predicted. It appears that removing food and water from a hopelessly comatose patient is a substantially more agoniz-

Table 20.1

Sample Living Will from Virginia Statutes

§54-325.8:4. *Suggested Form of Written Declaration.* A declaration executed pursuant to this article may, but need not, be in the following form, and may include other specific directions including, but not limited to, a designation of another person to make the treatment decision for the declarant should he be (i) diagnosed as suffering from a terminal condition and (ii) comatose, incompetent or otherwise mentally or physically incapable of communication. Should any other specific directions be held to be invalid, such invalidity shall not affect the declaration.

Declaration made this ＿＿＿ day of ＿＿＿＿＿ (month, year). I, ＿＿＿＿＿＿＿＿＿＿ , willfully and voluntarily make known my desire that my dying shall not be artificially prolonged under the circumstances set forth below, and do hereby declare:

If at any time I should have a terminal condition and my attending physician has determined that there can be no recovery from such condition and my death is imminent, where the application of life-prolonging procedures would serve only to artificially prolong the dying process, I direct that such procedures be withheld or withdrawn, and that I be permitted to die naturally with only the administration of medication or the performance of any medical procedure deemed necessary to provide me with comfort and care or to alleviate pain.

In the absence of my ability to give directions regarding the use of such life-prolonging procedures, it is my intention that this declaration shall be honored by my family and physician as the final expression of my legal right to refuse medical or surgical treatment and accept the consequences of such refusal.

I understand the full import of this declaration and I am emotionally and mentally competent to make this decision.

＿＿＿＿＿＿＿＿＿＿＿＿＿ (Signed)

The declarant is known to me and I believe him or her to be of sound mind. (1983, c. 532.)

＿＿＿＿＿＿＿＿＿＿＿＿　　　　　　＿＿＿＿＿＿＿＿＿＿＿＿

Witness　　　　　　　　　　　　　　　*Witness*

ing and controversial decision than removing medical-treatment machines.

Remaining Questions

There are many questions yet to be confronted: Is nourishment administered through an intravenous or other feeding tube "extraordinary care"? Will limiting governmental and private health-insurance benefits cause physicians and hospital personnel to coerce families to decide to refuse life-sustaining procedures for the patient? Will the exercise of the incompetent's "right to die" be made by families with improper motives, such as a desire to remarry, to inherit the patient's estate, or to avoid personal financial loss from the cost of the patient's care? Will the terminally ill retain the right to receive extraordinary care if that is his desire? Will the right to die continue to be an individual's personal choice imposed on society, or will the "right to die" become society's choice imposed on the individual?

In summary, it must be remembered that the incompetent person depends on the law and lawgivers to establish his rights when he is unable to act for himself. The court's traditional role has been to protect the incompetent and to consider his best interest, regardless of the cross-currents of societal controversy engendered by a specific situation. The admonition of the Supreme Judicial Court of Massachusetts, as enunciated in its opinion, in the case of *In Re Saikewicz*, continues to be the basis for consideration of the incompetent's fate:

> It does not advance the interest of the State or the ward to treat the ward as a person of lesser status or dignity than others. To protect the incompetent person within its power, the State must recognize the dignity and worth of such a person and afford to that person the same panoply of rights and choices it recognizes in competent persons.

Glossary

attorney-in-fact an individual (not necessarily an attorney-at-law) appointed by another (referred to as the "principal") to act on the principal's behalf either for some particular purpose, as to do a particular act, or for the transaction of business in general. The authority is conferred by an instrument in writing called a "letter of attorney," or more commonly, a "power of attorney."

conservator a guardian; protector; preserver. One who is appointed by a court to manage the estate of a protected person.

extraordinary care medical treatment that, under the circumstances of the patient's condition, may be deemed medically futile.

guardian a person lawfully invested with the power, and charged with the duty, of taking care of the person and managing the property and rights of another person, who, for defect of age, understanding, or self-control, is considered incapable of administering his own affairs.

informed consent before the patient may consent to the administration or withholding of medical treatment, the patient must receive all the facts available upon which to make an intelligent decision. In addition, the patient must be competent or the person rendering the consent has the authority to act on behalf of the patient.

medical feasibility consideration of the risk of harm to the patient from the administration of medical treatment weighed against the potential benefit to the patient.

right to die a right exercised by a competent person or by an individual having the authority to act on behalf of an incompetent person to refuse life-sustaining medical treatment. The authority of a legal representative to exercise this right varies from state to state.

References

Malcolm, A. H. 1986. "Reassessing care of dying: policy seen evolving from AMA opinion." *New York Times*, 16 March.

Myers, D. W. 1981, 1985. *Medico-legal implications of death and dying*. Rochester, N.Y.: The Lawyers Cooperative Publishing Co.; and San Francisco, Calif.: Bancroft Whitney Co.; and cumulative supplements.

Wallas, C. 1986. "To feed or not to feed." *Time*, Medicare Section, 31 March.

PART IV

Directions

Alzheimer's Disease and Related Disorders Association: Birth and Evolution of a Major Voluntary Health Association

Nancy E. Lombardo, Ph.D.

Past: Birth and Beyond

IN THE FALL OF 1979, THE necessary conditions for formation of a national Alzheimer's disease (AD) organization were in place. First, in leading major medical centers across the country, and most importantly, the National Institutes of Health (NIH) and National Institute of Mental Health (NIMH) in Washington, D.C., it had been recognized that AD was in fact the major cause of so-called senility in people over the age of sixty-five and that it affected well over two million Americans. Researchers in these places understood that AD was the proper diagnosis for the majority of dementia cases, not "hardening of the arteries," "organic brain syndrome," or "brain atrophy," as had previously been believed. Hitherto, the medical world held the mistaken belief that AD was an uncommon illness affecting fewer than a hundred thousand adults in their fifties and early sixties.

This new medical knowledge resulted from research conducted in England and the United States in the sixties and early seventies and which, by the late seventies, was becoming accepted in leading medical centers and universities across the country. The most important consequence of that research was the realization that, with increasing numbers of people living into their seventies and eighties, when AD is most prevalent, the number of Alzheimer patients was expected to grow very rapidly in the next few decades.

Second, in 1978 and 1979, at least seven independent local organizations—in Boston, Columbus, Minneapolis, New York City, Pittsburgh, Seattle, and San Francisco—had been created in response to local needs for more action in the realm of AD or other dementias. A meeting of the seven local groups was called by the NIH in Washington, D.C., in October 1979. Dr. Robert Butler, then director of the National Institute on Aging (NIA), initiated the meeting with Drs. John Tower and Katherine Bick of the National Institute of Neurological Diseases, Communicative Disorders and Strokes.

Robert Butler recognized the magnitude of the problems AD portended for society as well as the heartache and personal tragedies it represented for its victims and their families. As head of the NIA he felt a sense of responsibility to increase public awareness of AD, but he believed that this could be achieved only through a citizen- or lay-based group, a voluntary health association. He understood that new medical knowledge spreads rather slowly when dependent on only doctors, researchers, and government bureaucrats for its dissemination. When concerned citizens who feel a sense of personal urgency and who can reach out into every sector of American life get involved in spreading the news, information dissemination can be remarkably quick.

At the October 1979 meeting, the seven groups agreed to join together with a handful of other dedicated individuals, and the national organization was born, christened the

"Alzheimer's Disease and Related Disorders Association" (ADRDA). A critical ingredient from the beginning was the presence of a gifted leader, Jerome H. Stone, of Chicago, who challenged the group and himself to guarantee the first year's budget of $78,000. An initial board of directors was created, and an election of officers was held at a subsequent meeting. Stone was elected president (now chairman) and Lonnie Wollin, of New York City, treasurer, positions still held by these founders. ADRDA was formally created as a legal entity when Articles of Incorporation were filed in April 1980 and bylaws were adopted by the new national board of directors at a meeting in Chicago in June 1980.

The new organization had as its charge four major goals: increased public awareness and education, stimulation of research toward finding the cause and a cure, providing support for families, and stimulating advocacy and public policy.

The new organization was comprised of diverse interests, all of which are still represented on the national board of directors, which is the governing board of the association. The association itself is comprised of its member chapters. The national directors are elected from three constituencies: the member chapters elect up to twenty regional delegates, the Medical and Scientific Advisory Board designates four of its members as their representatives, and the board collectively elects other members at large, termed "public board members," who have traditionally been either persons of substance who could contribute their name or wealth to the association or major contributors of time and talent to ADRDA. The board currently consists of business, civic, and professional leaders from throughout the country, elected by their peers, the majority of whom are family members.

Progress

The level of energy, determination, talent, and effectiveness of the leaders of this national movement is unusually high, perhaps because many have a deep commitment motivated by personal tragedy and a sense of urgency. The result has been rapid progress on many fronts in the first seven years of ADRDA's existence.

The national organization has grown from a board of directors of ten people to the current occupancy of sixty-four board members, including twenty delegates representing chapters, four elected by the Medical and Scientific Advisory Board, and forty public board members.

The national budget for the organization doubled or tripled in the beginning years. The national budget for 1980 was $78,000, $250,000 in 1981, $650,000 in 1982, $1.5 million in 1983, $2.2 million in 1984, $4.1 million in 1985, $6.5 million in 1986, and $9.8 million in 1987.

For the first several months, ADRDA had no paid staff. A one-desk office was opened in New York City in 1980 and a national newsletter was published. The Association began to have the capabilities to respond to AD family members' information needs. In September 1981, the national headquarters office was opened in Chicago, and the Association's first executive director was hired.

While much of the work of ADRDA is still performed by volunteers, ADRDA paid staff has grown significantly and now handles the bulk of day-to-day work of running the organization at the national level with liaison to all chapters. Currently, ADRDA's national headquarters staff consists of sixty-five people plus volunteers, and the majority of ADRDA chapters employ staff to work in conjunction with their volunteers.

The national ADRDA is formally comprised of its member chapters. The number of chapter members of ADRDA has been increasing at a steady pace: there were fifteen chapters at the end of the first year and sixty-six active chapters at the 3½-year mark, for an average growth rate of nineteen new chapters per year. There were eighty-seven chapters in January 1984, when the board devised an experimental new category of affiliation, the "affiliate," and many new groups chose this category as a less demanding alternative. (This designation was discontinued in October 1986.) By January 1, 1986, there were 125 chapters and affiliates; after January 9, 1986, there were 143 groups, 110 chapters and 33 affiliates; currently, there are 176 chapters and affiliates in 46 states, which represents an average growth rate of twenty-two or twenty-three chapters and affiliates per year. In addition, the national ADRDA and its member chapters have fostered and encouraged the growth of over one thousand Alzheimer family support groups.

The chapter program had become increasingly complex over the seven-year period of ADRDA's growth. Initially, all new chapter development work was done by two volunteers, Bobbie Glaze, soon joined by Hilda Pridgeon, in Minnesota, who used the telephone, mails, and personal visits to encourage groups all over the United States to join ADRDA. Bobbie Glaze was appointed the first chairman of the then Program Development Committee (later Chapter Development Committee and then simply Chapter Committee); soon she had a committee of chapter representatives from all over the country. In late 1981, the first staff person for Chapters was hired. The Chapter Committee now has five subcommittees totaling over fifty volunteers to handle all the board-related business. Hiring of chapter staff has been given high priority, and currently the Association employs twelve field and office staff, under the direction of a vice-president.

Nearly five hundred thousand people, most of them representing AD families, receive the national newsletter, and additional thousands receive local chapter literature and newsletters.

The chapters provide community-level programs for ADRDA in the four areas of patient and family services, education, public policy, and research. Chapters provide families with basic information about the disease and how to cope with its myriad difficulties and devastating experiences, chapter support group meetings and hotlines to provide person-to-person mutual support and "how-to" information and encouragement, and referrals to existing patient-care services. Chapters also provide programs in education and public awareness, including speakers bureaus, newsletters, and general informational meetings. And as we shall learn presently, local chapters have been key in nationally organized public policy advocacy and public-awareness campaigns, and to a more variable degree, helpful in raising funds for research. The newest area of program activity for both the national office and local chapters is in the field of patient services, especially respite-care services and patient and family counseling. The national organization has initiated a National Demonstration Respite Care Program, which attempts to identify the most effective models for these programs.

It has been a natural evolution for many chapters to become involved with public policy. Therefore, state-level task forces on AD and legislation to benefit patients and families have been promulgated in more than 30 states. The Board of Directors also has authorized five state organizations to facilitate a coordinated approach to issues affecting Alzheimer families.

Alzheimer's Disease International (ADI)

In October 1984, ADRDA launched Alzheimer's Disease International (ADI) by calling a meeting in Washington, D.C., with the encouragement of the World Health Organization, and invited representatives from England, Canada, and Australia, which already had grass-roots-level Alzheimer organizations, and Belgium, France, and Germany, where individuals hoped one day to create a national Alzheimer society. In September 1985, the first European meeting of ADI was held in Belgium, and the second European meeting was held in Paris in September 1986. Each meeting was very successful and helped launch or strengthen new national Alzheimer organizations in Belgium, France, the Netherlands, Germany, and elsewhere. Princess Yasmin Aga Khan, who is a vice-chairman of ADRDA, was elected president of ADI in 1984. The vice-presidents include two other Americans who are also vice-chairmen of ADRDA, Ethan A. Hitchcock and Mrs. George F. Berlinger, and Canadian, Australian, and Belgian representatives.

The Present: Meeting Our Goals

EDUCATION AND PUBLIC AWARENESS

The dramatic increase in public awareness regarding AD during the last several years is perhaps the primary achievement of ADRDA to date. It lays the groundwork for future progress toward all of its other objectives.

Four years ago very few Americans had heard the phrase "Alzheimer's disease," let alone knew what it meant. Today, largely as a result of ADRDA's efforts, millions of Americans know about AD from their friends, neighbors, and relatives, from local and national newspapers and magazines, and from radio and TV reports, news specials, and documentaries, including the well-received "Do You Remember Love," starring Joanne Woodward and Richard Kiley.

Increased public awareness and deliberate outreach and education of health professionals by ADRDA and its member chapters and advisory board members have already had a profound effect on the medical and nonmedical care and treatment of Alzheimer patients. Almost every major medical and health professional journal and convention has featured AD in the last five years. Physicians and other health professionals are becoming more aware of the nature and importance of this disease. Increasing numbers of persons over the age of sixty-five are now receiving the correct diagnosis of "probable Alzheimer's disease" instead of meaningless or incorrect labels such as "hardening of the arteries," "chronic organic brain syndrome," or simply "senility." More and more physicians are being asked to take the condition seriously and attempt to manage the care of the patient rather than dismissing the family and patient by saying, "He [or she] is simply getting old, and there's nothing you can do about it."

The ADRDA experience is an example of the fact that new medical knowledge can be spread throughout an entire society, including the majority of physicians, much more rapidly by an active national grass-roots consumer movement than by medical, scientific, and government leaders acting on their own.

Five to ten years ago there was virtually no written information available to the lay public, and not much more was available to the health-care community about AD, whether on the details about the progression of the illness and its symptoms or on how a caregiver should manage the patient. Currently, a variety of materials exists on these issues, so that Alzheimer families have access to a vast reservoir of information.

RESEARCH

The quantity and quality of research activity related to AD and related disorders have increased dramatically in the last several years, although the total dollar value (e.g., $17 million in the fiscal year 1982 for NIH-sponsored research) is a drop in the bucket compared to the estimated $26 billion spent on care for current victims ($14 billion on nursing-home care alone, with an additional $12 billion spent on twice as many patients living at home). In 1982, the $26-billion figure did not include economic costs related to job loss of the patient or caregiver. Less than one-thousandth of total health-care costs is spent on research.

The national ADRDA has already been successful in encouraging the NIH and Congress to increase appropriations for NIH-sponsored Alzheimer basic research to $22.3 million for the fiscal year 1983, to $25 million in the 1984 budget, to nearly $50 million in fiscal year 1986, and to $65 million in fiscal year 1987. The national ADRDA has directly added to research support by awarding nineteen small research grants to help investigators qualify for larger NIH grants. In April 1983, ADRDA authorized its first faculty research program and also awarded two grants to existing AD brain banks, with authorization for a third in 1986. Currently, ADRDA's budget for research is $2.2 million. The family support group chapter network has been utilized by the national Medical and Scientific Advisory Board to establish an Autopsy Network. The Autopsy Network provides information and help to families seeking to arrange autopsy of victims for either diagnostic or research purposes. The board set aside $50,000 in funds to be distributed by chapters to give financial assistance to needy families in paying for autopsies.

PUBLIC POLICY

Public policy concerning AD, as with American health policy in general, is made in many locations, with many participants. Public policy-making is a slow process, and the changes desired by ADRDA will likely take a long time to achieve. Relevant policies and decisions are made in a myriad of institutions, within Congress, in several different government agencies, and in state legislatures and governmental departments in each of fifty states as well as among the major health-insurance carriers and their policyholders (particularly unions). The nation's medical centers, hospitals, nursing homes, and every other private and public health-care agency and many individual health-care providers play a part in deciding which services to offer, to whom, the quality of care, which patients are seen, and how they are treated.

ALZHEIMER FAMILIES
FIND EACH OTHER

Prior to the emergence of ADRDA and its component chapters and related support groups, Alzheimer patients and their families were isolated and usually silent, thinking their patient had a "rare" disease. Problems connected with the care of "senile" spouses, parents, or grandparents were hidden from view, as many families were too embarrassed to seek assistance. Many patients were also mislabeled or misdiagnosed as having mental illness, especially when patients suffered hallucinations, paranoia, or depression. With such a range of terms used, families of patients with the same disease(s) did not know they were dealing with the same or similar illnesses. Most families who sought medical information or help were unsuccessful and eventually gave up. Feeling alone, many were discouraged from even asking for better services, financing, or more research.

Researchers and medical leaders who established that AD was the cause of the majority of dementia cases made the first contribution to recognition of common interests among families. This in turn led to the formation of support groups and the national ADRDA. The public awareness achievements of ADRDA have meant that hundreds of thousands of families now recognize their common interests and realize that millions of people are afflicted.

ADRDA has already had significant political achievements for such a young organization. The first National Alzheimer's Disease Week was approved by Congress and proclaimed by the President for Thanksgiving week 1982. Not only was the Alzheimer's Public Awareness Week a big public rela-

the government is reducing both funded services and government insurance coverage (both Medicare and Medicaid).

It has been noted by a member of the Public Policy Committee that the current crisis in health-care costs "has led to a raising of insurance premiums, limitations in coverage, and a search for cost containment. At the same time, our patients live longer because of the advances made in medical science in curing or treating formerly fatal disease." Unless there are specialized programs targeted to AD and related disorders, there will soon be fewer, not more, resources available to combat AD and assist patients and families.

Just as the ADRDA national organization has begun to develop an ability to influence public policy on a national level—working with both the government agencies and Congress—the power over many key items of concern to families is being transferred to the states. Decision making in the health-care arena is already very dispersed; it is becoming even more decentralized under the New Federalism, with more authority regarding Medicaid and other key matters becoming state controlled. Currently, ADRDA is bringing to state legislatures the same concerns already brought to the national Congress, and a majority of states have now convened AD task forces or identified Alzheimer legislative efforts.

We've come a long way, but we've got still further to go. While we have succeeded in increasing awareness, we have reached only a small percentage of AD families. The situation is compounded by the fact that there are more than 300,000 new patients diagnosed every year, according to Hay and Ernst. In addition, we must make sure that the term "Alzheimer's disease" is not used before a careful medical evaluation has been performed.

While we've stimulated new research efforts and while new advances are made quite frequently, we still do not know the cause of this dreaded disease, and we have no cure. The dollar amount committed to Alzheimer research is infinitesimal in relation to the dollars spent on care, and there must be an increase in the resources available for research.

Families have learned that they can count on ADRDA for information about the disease itself, about services that may be available, and about policy and programs that might affect their well-being. And some families find ADRDA support groups a lifeline. Additionally, ADRDA continues to fight Alzheimer's disease on all fronts, including medical and scientific issues, continuing education, and research.

Government officials and policymakers are becoming increasingly aware of the plight of Alzheimer victims and families, especially as regards the need for long-term care. We need sweeping changes regarding the financing of such services. This issue is currently of high priority with the Association and is a focus of national legislative activity.

ADRDA is a remarkable organization whose growth and achievements have been exemplary. Looking to the future, ADRDA has a full agenda and will need to continue its unprecedented multifaceted efforts on behalf of AD victims and their families.

References

Hay, J., and Ernst, R. 1987. Economic costs of Alzheimer's disease. *Am. J. Public Health* 77:9, 1169–75.

U.S. Congress, Office of Technology Assessment. April 1987. *Losing a million minds: confronting the tragedy of Alzheimer's disease and other dementias.* Washington, D.C.: U.S. Government Printing Office.

CHAPTER TWENTY-TWO

Legislative Advocacy and Alzheimer's Disease: Facing the Future, Meeting the Needs

Kathryn C. Rees, M.A.

ALZHEIMER'S DISEASE (AD) IS receiving increased attention at all levels of government due to the rising social and economic impact associated with the disease; the tremendous burdens placed on the families afflicted; and the political activism of the Alzheimer's Disease and Related Disorders Association (ADRDA) and its families.

The "National Program to Conquer Alzheimer's Disease," the legislative goals statement, has played a key role in the design of each state's advocacy objectives. California, for example, has been a leader in Alzheimer advocacy, and a variety of legislative initiatives have been passed since 1984 that have established the foundation on which future programs will be built. These measures were in the following areas: task forces/study groups, diagnosis, and treatment; research; respite; entitlements; and insurance. While we have

337

succeeded in carving out a place in the legislative and social agendas, we are still far from meeting the needs of many Alzheimer families.

Task Forces/Study Groups

Initially, to help identify and prioritize the needs of Alzheimer victims and families, the California legislature passed ADRDA-supported legislation creating an Alzheimer's Disease Task Force. Its mandates included convening a state-wide conference on AD and proposing options to the governor and the state legislature regarding the expansion of existing programs and development of new ones. A task-force approach is particularly useful in legitimizing, in the eyes of public officials, the need for services so critical to Alzheimer families and in setting the stage for subsequent legislation. A number of other states, for example, Illinois, Maryland, Michigan, Massachusetts, Ohio, Virginia, and New Jersey, have passed similar legislation, establishing a task force or advisory-committee study group to analyze the problems raised by AD and to recommend appropriate action. It is the hope of ADRDA that all other states will understand the necessity of such task forces and adopt their own measures.

Diagnosis and Treatment

Recognizing the need for an accurate diagnosis of AD, California established six Alzheimer's Disease Diagnostic and Treatment Centers at six University of California medical centers. The centers provide a complete diagnostic workup for Alzheimer patients, offer a wide variety of planning and support activities for family members, and work to help increase the level of education and training of health-care professionals. The diagnostic and treatment centers are pilot projects whose future existence still needs to be secured. In New Jersey, the legislature provided funding for a diagnostic and treatment center. In Massachusetts, a diagnostic center was created in Worcester. Ohio has provided funds for diagnostic services.

Furthermore, research became part of the state legislative agenda, although admittedly at a modest level ($750,000 total for fiscal year 1986–87). The California chapter's decision to pursue state-sponsored research funding, in addition to major efforts occurring at the federal level, was based on the fact that areas currently receiving little attention at the federal level are those that impact the most on state and local funding levels: early and accurate detection of the disease, management and treatment of patients, reducing care costs, and disease prevention. Other states have appropriated funds to expand research efforts. Illinois was the first state to list an Alzheimer's Disease Research Fund as an optional contribution—or "checkoff"—if a refund was due to a taxpayer. The state's local ADRDA chapters worked closely with the Department of Public Health to raise public awareness of this voluntary checkoff on the 1985 forms; approximately $115,000 already raised for the fund will be earmarked for new Alzheimer researchers.

Respite

Like research, expanded funding for respite care is of the highest priority. Even when families have the means to purchase respite care, the services are often unavailable. The ability to provide relief to the caregiver is often the difference between the patient's remaining at home or being placed in an institution. The state of California has achieved only modest results in this area. In 1986 the legislature passed two bills that established respite-care registries, which will identify needs, make referrals to existing respite-care projects, and report to the legislature on the types of services provided, the number of services needed but unavailable, and the effectiveness of respite care in delaying institutionalization. It is hoped that the studies will provide the data necessary to establish comprehensive, publicly funded respite-care programs.

Additionally, legislation was passed establishing a three-year demonstration project permitting general acute-care hospitals and nursing homes to utilize empty beds to provide temporary respite services for frail elderly, functionally impaired, and mentally disordered adults. Other states, including Connecticut, Delaware, Florida, Hawaii, and New Jersey, have provided funding to create specialized respite-and/or day-care programs. Massachusetts has allocated funds for a state hospital to design a specialized Alzheimer unit, and the state's Veterans Administration system has initiated special care for Alzheimer patients.

In 1984 legislation was passed in California creating a three-year pilot project of eight Alzheimer's Day Care Resource Centers. These centers are to provide a spectrum of services for Alzheimer patients and their families, including respite care, day care, support services, assessment, information and referral, and training for caregivers. Future goals include the continuation and expansion of these special models of care for Alzheimer patients. Other states, including Massachusetts, New Jersey, Ohio, and Maryland, have also established day- and respite-care initiatives.

In 1984, the California Department of Health Services initiated a Preadmission Screening Pilot Program with hospitals and nursing homes to determine the appropriate placement of patients referred to skilled nursing facilities, whether from general acute-care hospitals or from the community. The screening process was developed to determine the proper site for placement of the patient, the needed level of care, and the availability of appropriate community-based services. This process addresses two major concerns: The first issue is to help reduce the high costs of long-term institutional care by referring patients, where medically appropriate, to less costly community-based services, such as social and adult day care and respite care. Second, this service will be valuable in identifying available community-based services to Alzheimer families who wish to keep their relative at home, in the least restrictive environment, for as long as possible.

The initial pilot program has already been expanded to operate statewide and has been directed to report to the legislature on the number of persons diverted to community-based services, and the number of persons unable to be diverted and why, including personal choice, medical condition, and the lack of community-based supportive services. Thus, a data base will be built to support the need for increased community-based supportive services and will simultaneously be available to educate families on the availability of services in their area.

Entitlements

Numerous legal problems plague families facing AD (see chapters 18, 19, and 20). Critical choices must be made regarding finances, health care, and personal matters for a family member whose functional capabilities are deteriorating.

California families were greatly concerned by the problems caused by the impoverishment of one spouse when the other was institutionalized. This situation occurred because of the "spend-down" requirement for Medicaid (Medi-Cal) eligibility. Couples were sometimes forced to divorce to prevent the noninstitutionalized spouse from being driven into poverty.

In response to these concerns, legislation in California was passed to address the division of community property of a married couple for the purposes of Medicaid (Medi-Cal) eligibility. The bill mandated that the state amend its rules to automatically divide the community property of a married couple in half, making the noninstitutionalized spouse's property unavailable for consideration for Medicaid (Medi-Cal) eligibility for nursing-home placement. Kansas has similar legislation in process.

Lawmakers have the delicate task of creating public policy that is balanced between protecting individual rights and providing families and professionals with the flexibility to make decisions that are in the best interests of the patient. California has recently passed legislation that requires that public conservators place conservatees in the least restrictive setting as close to home as possible.

Financing and Insurance Issues

Financing problems are a critical concern for Alzheimer patients and their families. Many are often impoverished by this long-term illness. Families have frequently raised the question of some financial relief in the form of tax credits or tax deductions.

The California legislature has been attempting to pass some form of tax relief legislation since 1984. While there seems to be a genuine interest in the concept, the measures have died. However, the governor recently indicated a willingness to consider tax deductions for respite care, but no legislation has yet been passed. In South Carolina, a bill has passed allowing a nonrefundable, limited state-income-tax credit for expenses paid by the taxpayer to an intermediate- or skilled-care facility. With federal, state, and local governments facing dwindling fiscal resources, lawmakers are turning to the private sector to provide leadership in developing models of financial relief for overburdened caregivers.

There has been a flurry of activity regarding the financing of long-term care. Several states (e.g., Colorado, Washington, West Virginia) have passed legislation that encourages long-term-care coverage for AD; others, including Texas and Kansas, have authorized studies.

Legislation was passed in California mandating a study of the feasibility of long-term-care insurance coverage. The Department of Insurance is required to submit a report to the legislature by July 1, 1988, to include a study of public policy initiatives that will encourage the development of private long-term-care insurance; educational initiatives to inform the public on the need for long-term-care insurance that covers both institutional and home-based care; and directives on how the government and private industry can work together to protect individuals against the high costs of long-term care. Studies of this nature help to build a data base that can be used to support the introduction of new programs.

Education and training initiatives have taken many forms, including a statewide education and training center in Georgia; training for family caregivers in Iowa; in-service education for personnel in institutions and sheltered housing in Maryland; an information clearinghouse in Pennsylvania; and physician training in Ohio.

Future Trends

While the expansion of services under government entitlement programs is extremely important, the current conservative trend in our country and constitutional limits on spending in many states may limit major achievements in this area in the near future. In California, and, in fact, nationally, we would anticipate a strong push in the areas of research, respite care, expansion of community-based services, diagnosis and treatment, and development of insurance coverage. Additionally, we cannot ignore the increasing interest in development of sweeping public policy reforms in the financing of health and long-term care.

In addition to existing programs, lawmakers are seeking to develop creative methods of providing services. In California, among the programs to be studied is a credit-service plan whereby healthy seniors would volunteer to provide in-home care for the frail and functionally impaired elderly. In return, they would accrue "credit" for hours worked, to be used should they or a friend or relative need the service. Programs of this nature are thought to be relatively inexpensive to administer while simultaneously providing opportunities for healthy senior citizens to participate in the caring process.

Additional directions in education and training would include curricular expansion in medical, nursing, law, and social-work schools to include instruction on dementia and its effects. Staff members working with Alzheimer victims in any setting will need to receive specialized training, with content appropriate to their roles.

Your Role in the Political Process

You, as a family member or other interested person, need to be aware that Alzheimer victims and their families are excluded in many ways from our health-care and social-service delivery systems. Advocacy efforts have been strong and successful at local and state levels; however, more uniform and better programs must be developed as part of a *national* health-care plan that includes Alzheimer victims and their families. Future progress will depend on the involvement of ADRDA members with both advocacy and public policy.

CHAPTER TWENTY-THREE

Research Directions in Alzheimer's Disease: Advances and Opportunities

Robert Katzman, M.D.

IN THE SPRING OF 1985, THE *New York Times* published the obituary of Sir Robert Meyer, who died at the age of 105. There is no doubt about Sir Robert Meyer's birth date. He was born in Germany and was a child prodigy who had been introduced to Brahms at the age of ten. However, he did not make it in the world of musical geniuses and in his late teens emigrated to Great Britain, where he entered into business, becoming so successful that he retired in 1923 a rich man and a philanthropist. He devoted his subsequent years to giving concerts for children in Great Britain. These became a tradition, and Queen Elizabeth and the current

This chapter is based on Katzman, R. 1987. Alzheimer's disease: advances and opportunities, *Journ. of the Amer. Ger. Soc.* 35:69–73. Reprinted with permission.

Prince of Wales were introduced to classical music through them. I had the opportunity to meet Sir Robert Meyer in 1980 when he visited the United States. He had just lectured to the Music Department at Sarah Lawrence College, after which a reception was held for him. During this reception he would move his wheelchair (he had just broken his hip, but no orthopedic surgeon in Great Britain would pin it because he was 100 years old) to a knot of people in conversation, demand to know what the subject was, and interact vigorously with them. The following day Sir Robert lectured at Princeton, the next day at Columbia, and finally he went to Washington, D.C., to meet with the Endowment for the Humanities, hoping to obtain additional funds for his concert series. I consider that Sir Robert epitomizes what we all ought to expect as normal aging.

Normal Aging Versus Dementia

Not all of us will be as fortunate as Sir Robert Meyer. A significant minority of older persons become demented due to disease processes that alter brain function. The two most important disease processes, Alzheimer's disease (AD) and multiple strokes—which together account for three-fourths of individuals with dementia—are both age-dependent disorders, occurring more frequently with increased age. However, the altered brain function is due to the presence of disease rather than to a normal aging process. Age-dependent diseases have risk factors, causes, and cures, as do diseases at any age. The best example is that of dementia due to stroke. The incidence of stroke in the United States has fallen about 50 percent during the past twenty years. Data prior to 1970 show that 2 percent of the population per year died at age eighty from stroke. In a prospective study of eighty-year-olds carried out in New York City, we found that the incidence of new cases of stroke from 1981 to 1984 was only 1.1 percent per year. No doubt this decrease in the occurrence of stroke is due to improved treatment of hypertension and adjustment of diet and life-style. Conceivably, the incidence may fall even further. With the advent of molecular genetics and the ability to produce blood components that dissolve clots, the era of treatment of stroke may be at hand. Thus, within our lifetime, we may see the occurrence of brain damage from stroke reduced to the point where it will become a rare condition.

Similar advances in prevention and treatment have not yet been achieved with AD. In fact, with the anticipated growth of the very elderly population, there is every reason to project a major increase in the number of Alzheimer victims in coming decades. The incidence of AD rises steeply from age sixty to at least age eighty-five. At age sixty, the incidence is less than .1 percent per year; at age eighty, the incidence is about 2 percent per year, or twenty times as high. When the declining death rate of the very old is considered and certain assumptions are made regarding the maximum incidence of AD and life expectancy of patients, it can be projected that approximately one-third of the population over ninety will have AD. As we succeed in reducing the death rate of the very elderly, we increase the population at greatest risk for this disorder. It will be difficult to keep pace with the needs of Alzheimer patients during the next fifty years, as the population over eighty-five years of age triples, unless research into the causes and treatment of AD becomes a priority and the number of severely impaired is reduced. Is there a reasonable chance that we may, in the next twenty years, learn enough about AD to begin to prevent or treat it? I believe so.

Describing the Disease

Alois Alzheimer initially described this disorder in 1906 and subsequently published his findings fully in 1907. Alzheimer's discovery was readily accepted, and by 1910 the condition he described was incorporated into Kraeplein's *Textbook of Psychiatry* as a presenile (under age sixty-five) dementia. This no doubt set the field back by many years, for during the next decades there was no agreement as to whether elderly individuals with dementia whose brains upon autopsy exhibited the structures Alzheimer described could be considered to have had AD. Further confusion was created by the belief, particularly widespread in the United States, that most cases of senile dementia were due to "hardening of the arteries."

It was not until the 1960s that the situation began to be clarified. During this decade Terry and Kidd described the ultrastructure of the neurofibrillary tangles and neuritic plaques and showed that these changes occurred identically in brains of affected fifty-five-year-olds and brains of eighty-five-year-olds. Corsellis and Tomlinson carefully autopsied a series of institutionalized patients who had died of dementia and found no evidence to suggest that symptoms of senile (over age sixty-five) dementia were associated with the degree of arteriosclerosis of the blood vessels to the brain. In 1968, Blessed, Tomlinson, and Roth published results of their classic clinical pathological study. Using both a mental-status examination and a functional evaluation to examine patients hospitalized for chronic care, these investigators were able to identify patients with dementia during life and correlate their scores on the mental-status and functional tests with the pathology at time of death. They demonstrated that the majority of patients with dementia showed changes typical of the Alzheimer brain and that the number of neuritic plaques present in several areas of the cerebral cortex correlated very well both with the mental-status score and with the functional evaluation. These investigators also found that in those patients with brain-tissue disease and dementia, dementia was present when there had been multiple strokes, such that more than 50–100 grams of cerebral hemisphere were destroyed, producing areas of dead or dying tissue called infarcts. Hence the term "multi-infarct dementia," as coined subsequently by Hachinski.

In Tomlinson's and other autopsy series of patients with dementia, it became apparent that AD was the major cause of dementia in the elderly, accounting for 50–65 percent of cases. In the very old, the degree of dementia was related to the degree of pathological changes, and the ultrastructural changes were identical to those in the younger patients. AD could be considered to be a single disorder regardless of age at onset. It was then apparent that AD could become a major and growing problem as the population aged. I had the opportunity of verbalizing this relationship first in 1974 and subsequently in a 1976 editorial in the *Archives of Neurology*. My colleague, Dr. Robert Terry, and I then approached Dr. Donald Tower, the director of the National Institute of Neurological and Communicative Disorders and Strokes (NINCDS), about the possibility of a National Institutes of Health (NIH)–sponsored conference on this disorder. The result was a workshop conference sponsored by three institutes: the National Institute on Aging (NIA), the NINCDS, and the National Institute of Mental Health (NIMH). Interest in AD was further awakened in 1976 by the discovery of an 80–90 percent reduction within the cerebral cortex and hippocampus of the Alzheimer brain of the acetylcholine biosynthetic enzyme, choline acetyltransferase, another indication of the specific pathology of this disease.

Research Advances

Since 1976, there has been a substantial acceleration of research on AD. Whereas a decade ago it was possible for a single reviewer to cover the important literature in the field, this is no longer true today. A computerized search of articles on the subject now averages more than 150 new titles per month. Significant research advances have also been made during the past several years in such diverse areas as the discovery of specific pathological and neurotransmitter changes in the Alzheimer brain and their correlation with cognitive deficits, the identification of the molecular constituents of the abnormal fibrous proteins, and perhaps most surprising, the advances made in the accuracy of clinical diagnosis.

It is the intent of this chapter to provide a broad outline of some of the advances in the field and some of the most exciting research priorities.

ASSESSING THE DAMAGE: WHICH NERVE CELLS ARE AFFECTED BY THE ALZHEIMER PROCESS?

Although the clinical manifestations of AD seem to indicate widespread brain involvement, the Alzheimer process appears to selectively affect specific nerve cells (neurons) (see fig. 23.1).

The neuronal system that has received most attention and is affected very early in the course of AD is the basal cholinergic projection system. This neuronal system is easily identified because the neurons composing it uniquely contain choline acetyltransferase (ChAT), the biosynthetic enzyme that enables these cells to form acetylcholine, a chemical used by them to transmit signals to other cells. The neurons of this system originate in the forebrain and project to the cerebral cortex and hippocampus. Terminals of these nerve cells make up part of the neuritic plaques (accumulations of degenerating nerve terminals surrounding a core of amyloid protein) characteristic of AD. There is already evidence that a disruption in this neuronal system is closely linked with AD. For example, brain biopsies obtained from Alzheimer patients within months after the onset of symptoms reveal that ChAT is reduced by as much as 40 percent in the cere-

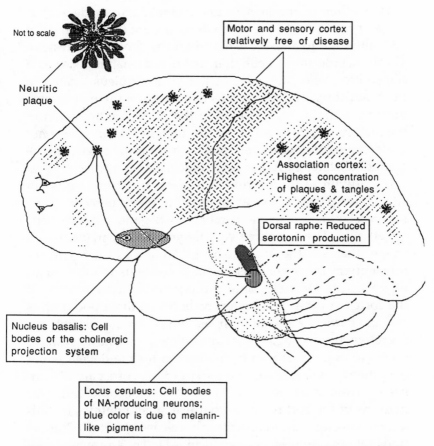

Not to scale

Motor and sensory cortex
relatively free of disease

Neuritic
plaque

Association cortex:
Highest concentration
of plaques & tangles

Dorsal raphe: Reduced
serotonin production

Nucleus basalis: Cell
bodies of the cholinergic
projection system

Locus ceruleus: Cell bodies
of NA-producing neurons;
blue color is due to melanin-
like pigment

Figure 23.1. Diagram showing the selective effects of AD on the brain. Although there appears to be widespread brain involvement, research reveals that only specific systems are involved.

bral cortex. Brain autopsies also reveal a reduction of ChAT in the hippocampus, which correlates well with Alzheimer patients' scores on mental-status and memory tests obtained up to eleven months before their death. Because of this evidence a number of investigators are searching for drugs that increase the activity of this system in order to provide some symptomatic relief to Alzheimer patients.

Two other neuronal systems projecting from deep portions of the brain to the cerebral cortex are also involved in AD, although to a lesser extent than the cholinergic system. These include nerve cells that use noradrenaline (NA) as a transmitter, cells that arise in the locus ceruleus located in the brain stem, and nerve cells that produce the neurotransmitter serotonin, cells located in the dorsal raphe region of the midbrain. Their role in the production of dementia is not understood, but serotonin plays an important part in the emotional states of AD patients, including depression.

In addition to these projection systems, brain autopsy of Alzheimer patients reveals that about 15–20 percent of the nerve cells located in the cerebral cortex and hippocampus degenerate. These include very large neurons, pyramidal in shape, that use the amino acid glutamate as their primary transmitter. These cells also form projections to other brain regions. Affected cells connect different association areas of the cortex or act as relay neurons between the hippocampus and the cortical association areas, which are responsible for cognitive processing. Thus involvement of these systems seems to imply that part of the reason for the development of dementia is that association areas of the cortex are disconnected from each other. In addition, some other intrinsic neurons of the cortex, those that use small peptides including somatostatin and corticotropin-releasing factor (CRF) as transmitters, are also destroyed in AD. Thus research, primarily through biopsy and autopsy, is beginning to construct a clearer picture of which cells are affected by the Alzheimer process, how they interconnect, and how dementia results.

PATTERNS OF CELLULAR DEGENERATION

AD involves a typical pattern of neuron degeneration that is marked microscopically by the presence of neurofibrillary tangles (abnormal nerve cell bodies) and neuritic plaques (see fig. 23.2). Other pathological hallmarks of AD include the

Neuritic Plaque (NP)

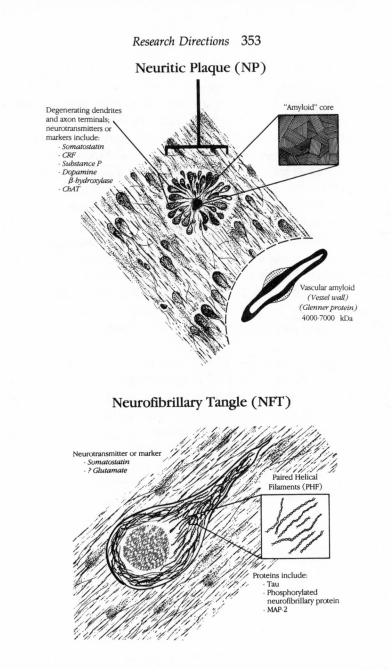

Neurofibrillary Tangle (NFT)

Figure 23.2. Diagrams showing a neuritic plaque (top) and a neurofibrillary tangle (bottom) and their components.

reduction in numbers of neurons in specific cell groups, the presence of degenerating granules and vacuoles in certain hippocampal neurons, and the presence of amyloid protein in some blood vessels of the cerebral cortex and its protective coverings. During the past two years researchers have isolated the major peptide found in cerebral blood vessel and neuritic plaque amyloid, identified its amino acid sequence, and found it to be a unique protein. The gene for the precursor to the amyloid protein (variously termed the beta amyloid peptide and the A4 protein) has been identified and its amino acid composition described. It is a gene present in normal individuals and is located on chromosome 21. There is now evidence that the position (locus) of the gene responsible for familial (hereditary) AD is on the same segment in chromosome 21. Whether there is a direct relationship between the familial AD gene and the A4 gene is not known at present.

Researchers have also made progress in identifying the protein constituents of neurofibrillary tangles and have found at least three proteins that help to form the skeleton of nerve cells (neuronal cytoskeleton). The complete structure of these tangles is not yet known. Thus some investigators consider AD to be a disease of the neuronal cytoskeleton, but the process by which these abnormalities occur is not yet understood.

ACCURACY OF DIAGNOSIS

Advances in clinical diagnostic accuracy have resulted from improved understanding of the presentation and course of the disease. In the 1970s, follow-up studies indicated an error rate of 30 percent or more in the diagnosis of AD, even in specialized referral centers such as the Maudsley Hospital in England. Clinical criteria for the diagnosis of dementia (e.g., those in the American Psychiatric Association's *Diagnostic and Statistical Manual of Mental Diseases*, 3rd ed.)

and AD (e.g., NINCDS and ADRDA) have now been developed that have greatly improved this situation. In the subgroup of patients who meet the clinical criteria of "probable Alzheimer's," about 90 percent have AD at postmortem examination. But clinical diagnosis is probably not as accurate in patients who meet criteria for "possible Alzheimer's," and we are not able to differentiate clinically patients with mixed AD and vascular dementia from patients with dementia caused by stroke alone. Clearly a specific test for AD remains an important priority.

Discovering Risk Factors via Cross-Cultural Studies

A useful approach that has led to identification of risk factors in other disorders has been the discovery of locales, groups, or cultures with a very high or very low incidence of a disease. So far such clues to risk factors in AD have not been forthcoming. Accurate clinical diagnosis has been achieved only recently and has had limited application; hence, ordinary sources of information, such as hospital records or death certificates, are questionable. If current diagnostic methods are to be used in other societies, mental-status and other verbal tests will not only need to be translated but also adapted for local culture; physicians will need to be trained in clinical criteria. Moreover, autopsy diagnosis, the most accurate form of diagnosis now possible, is carried out routinely in only a few Western countries. In the United States the autopsy rate in most hospitals is now below one-quarter of the deaths and about one-quarter of this rate for those in their seventies and beyond. In the Third World countries autopsies are rare. Also, if incidence between groups is to be compared, it must be age-specific incidence, as there is more than a twenty-fold rise in incidence between ages sixty and eighty-five. In many cultures, AD is considered to be either a natural age change in older individuals and therefore not reportable or a matter of shame to a family, as a result of which victims of the disease are hidden by the family. Thus, cross-cultural studies at present are difficult but need to be done.

BIOLOGIC MARKERS

Discovery of a specific biologic marker of AD in a body tissue such as skin, blood, or spinal fluid would have a profound impact both on clinical practice and on research into causes of the disorder. Diagnostic accuracy would increase especially in individuals with multiple diseases. A peripheral marker would make genetic studies much easier, and cross-cultural studies would become simpler to carry out.

Alternative Approaches to Treatment

TROPHIC FACTORS: CAN DISEASE PROGRESSION BE HALTED?

We now know that in normal development almost half of the nerve cells that are formed in the brain do not survive into adult life. This process of selective cell elimination ensures that only cells that have made appropriate connections survive; this process is no doubt involved in the "fine-tuning" of the brain's circuitry. In part, the determination of which cells survive appears to depend on specific proteins, known as trophic factors. Recently, evidence from animal experiments shows that one of the best-studied trophic factors, nerve growth factor (NGF), can act to promote survival of central-nervous-system neurons in adult life, acting fairly specifically on the septal cholinergic neurons, one of the classes of cells most involved in AD. Other known growth factors are capable of keeping hippocampal neurons alive in tissue culture. The question arises as to whether such factors could slow the death of these nerve cells in Alzheimer patients. This is an intriguing, although speculative, therapeutic approach.

BRAIN IMPLANTATION: CAN DEFICITS BE CORRECTED?

An exciting new tool in experimental neurology is the implantation of groups of nerve cells into the adult brain. One can identify a group of very elderly rats, constituting perhaps 20 percent of rats over the age of twenty-four months, who have difficulty running mazes. If neurons from fetal rat brain are transplanted into the hippocampus of these impaired rats, their ability to learn mazes is restored. Moreover, one can demonstrate histologically and neurophysiologically that the implanted cells have formed connections in a quite appropriate fashion with the existing hippocampal tissue. Whether this approach can be adapted to primates and humans is yet to be determined. However, a new source of these cells—for example, tissue culture (in which individual tissue cells are cultured in laboratory dishes to produce a crop of cells available for transplant)—will be needed because of the potential ethical and practical difficulties in using human fetal brain.

The medical and scientific communities have clearly made progress in their concerted effort to find the cause and develop treatment both for the disease itself and for its cognitive symptoms, particularly memory loss. The recent breakthroughs in basic research and the promising results of experimental drug treatment offer new hope to AD patients and their families as we continue the quest for the eradication of this illness.

Suggested Resources

Books and Periodicals

Note to the Reader: Items with an asterisk preceding the entry may be available through your local chapter of Alzheimer's Disease and Related Disorders Association or by contacting the national office of ADRDA for information.

GENERAL REFERENCES

*Aronson, M. K., and Jarvik, L., eds. Winter 1984. Alzheimer's update. *Generations (J. of the Western Ger. Soc.),* vol. 9.

An entire issue of the *Journal of the Western Gerontological Society,* devoted to the latest in research and caregiving.

*———, and Katzman, R., eds. Fall 1982. Alzheimer's disease and related disorders. *Generations,* vol. 7.

An earlier issue of the *J. of the Western Ger. Soc.* provides an overview of Alzheimer's disease, touching on diagnostic, legal, and caregiving issues.

Cohen, D., and Eisdorfer, C., 1986. *Loss of self.* New York: W. W. Norton Co.

An up-to-date, comprehensive resource for the friends and family of AD patients. A practical and readable guide that covers every aspect of the disease, illustrated with personal accounts of caregiving.

*Gwyther, L. 1985. *Care of Alzheimer patients: a manual for nursing home staff.* American Health Care Association and Alzheimer's Disease and Related Disorders Association.

A practical approach to hands-on care. Although geared to nursing aides, this manual may be helpful to family caregivers as well.

*Heston, L. L., and White, J. A. 1983. *Dementia—a practical guide to Alzheimer's disease.* New York: W. H. Freeman and Co.

This book demystifies the medical aspects of AD, with a lucid explanation of the diagnostic process and a particularly strong section on genetics.

Holland, G. B. 1985. *For Sasha, with love: an Alzheimer's crusade.* New York: Red Dembner Enterprises Corp.

A spouse describes her wrenching experience of caring for her demented husband. This book describes the ordeal and frustrations, as well as personal triumphs, of caring for an AD patient.

Kushner, H. S. 1981. *When bad things happen to good people.* New York: Schocken Books.

Inspirational advice on coping with the devastating effect of illness on loved ones.

*Mace, N. L., and Rabins, P. V. 1981. *The 36-Hour Day.* Baltimore: The Johns Hopkins University Press.

A useful guide to the practical problems of coping with the mental and physical impairments of Alzheimer patients. Offers tips on everything from dealing with catastrophic reactions to bathing the patient.

Matsuyama, S. S., and Jarvik, L. F. 1987. *Alzheimer Disease and Associated Disorders—An International Journal.* Law-

rence, Kans.: Western Geriatric Research Institute.
A new journal that is devoted solely to aspects of Alzheimer's disease and related disorders.

Office of Technology Assessment. 1987. *Losing a million minds: confronting the tragedy of Alzheimer's disease and other dementias.* Washington, D.C.: U.S. Government Printing Office.
An overview of Alzheimer's disease and implications for public policy. This report was published by Congress as a result of its concern for the plight of Alzheimer's disease patients and their families.

Roach, M. 1985. *Another name for madness.* Boston: Houghton Mifflin Co.
This is a dramatic story of one family's struggle with AD as told by the patient's daughter. Provides an insight into how one family came to terms with the devastating impact of Alzheimer's disease.

Sacks, O. 1985. *The man who mistook his wife for a hat.* New York: Summit Books.
Through case studies, this book explores a variety of neurological disorders and their effects on the minds and lives of those affected. A study of the struggle against extraordinary adversity.

Safford, F. 1986. *Caring for the mentally impaired elderly.* New York: Henry Holt and Co.
This book offers important advice on everything from diagnoses to death, based on the author's personal experience of working with families of dementia patients.

Swaab, D. F., Fliers, E., et al. 1986. *Progress in brain research, aging of the brain and Alzheimer's disease,* vol. 70. Elsevier Science Publishers.
A good resource for up-to-date scientific information.

Viorst, J. 1986. *Necessary losses.* New York; Simon and Schuster.
Presents a psychoanalytic view of life as a series of adap-

tations to loss, which may be used as a framework for dealing with Alzheimer's disease.

Choosing a nursing home for the person with intellectual loss. 1980. Burke Rehabilitation Center.
A guide to the issues one should address when considering nursing home placement.

The living will and other advance directives. 1986. New York: Concern for Dying.
A legal guide to medical treatment decisions. Discusses issues of legal competence and execution and enforcement of living wills, and provides advice to patients and their families.

ARTICLES

*Katzman, R. 1987. Alzheimer's disease: advances and opportunities. *J. of the Amer. Ger. Soc.* 35:69–73.

———. 1986. Medical progress: Alzheimer's disease. *New Eng. J. of Med.* 314:964–73.

Winograd, C. H., and Jarvik, L. F. 1986. Physician management of the demented patient. *J. of the Amer. Ger. Soc.* 34:295–308.

*Wurtman, R. J. 1985. Alzheimer's disease. *Scientific Amer.*, 252:62–66, 71–74.

BROCHURES/PERIODICALS

*AD *Newsletter*, published quarterly. Available through Alzheimer's Disease and Related Disorders Association.

*ADRDA brochure series on single topics, available through Alzheimer's Disease and Related Disorders Association.

Coping and caring: living with Alzheimer's disease, available through the American Association of Retired Persons (AARP), Washington, DC 20047.

FOR CHILDREN

*Guthrie, D. 1986. *Grandpa doesn't know it's me.* New York: Human Sciences Press.
A story portraying the progression of dementia in an elderly man from a child's point of view. Suitable for six- to nine-year-olds.

FOR TEENAGERS

Frank, J. 1985. *The silent epidemic.* Minneapolis: Lerner Publications Company.
An introduction to Alzheimer's disease through the story of a "typical" patient, enhanced by detailed diagrams and pictures. A clear description of what happens to the brain as the disease progresses and what causes the symptoms, geared to a young audience.

Films

Caring: Families Coping with Alzheimer's Disease
Do You Remember Love
Living with Grace
Someone I Once Knew
Whispering Hope
You Are Not Alone

Note: For most films, special license arrangements are in effect and distribution is restricted. Consult the national headquarters of ADRDA or your local ADRDA chapter for information.

Other Resources

Alzheimer's Disease and Related Disorders Association
70 E. Lake Street, Suite 600
Chicago, Illinois 60601
1-800-621-0379 or 1-800-572-6037 (in Illinois)

National Institute on Aging
NIA Information Center
2209 Distribution Circle
Silver Springs, Maryland 20910

Contributors

Harriet Adelstein, M.A., O.T.R., an occupational therapist, is a gerontologist, lecturer, consultant, trainer, and author. She has a private practice serving older adults and their families, is a cofounder of the Chicago chapter of ADRDA and has been an active member of the national ADRDA since it was founded. Mrs. Adelstein codeveloped and led the training program for lay leaders, the Second-Generation Program for ADRDA, a Chicago ADRDA support group for children and grandchildren of Alzheimer's disease patients. She is the author of *Educating Medical Professionals: A Manual for Lay Persons Planning and Implementing Training Programs on AD*.

Lesley Arshonsky, B.A., has an elementary-school teaching degree and has had extensive experience working with children and adolescents. She was instrumental in developing the concept of the Second-Generation Program, a Chicago ADRDA support group for children and grandchildren of Alzheimer's disease patients. Her father was diagnosed as having Alzheimer's disease at the age of fifty-four, and she saw the effects of this on her younger sister, who was still living at home. Mrs. Arshonsky is vice-president for fund-raising and development for the Chicago chapter of ADRDA.

Charles C. Bell, J.D., is a past vice-chairman of the public policy committee of the national ADRDA and an officer of its western

Pennsylvania chapter. Mr. Bell is an associate of the law firm of Hess, Reich, Georgiades, Ray, and Hornyak, P.C., in Pittsburgh, has written and lectured on various legal issues affecting victims of AD and their families.

JOHN C. S. BREITNER, M.D., M.P.H., is associate chief of staff for education at the Bronx Veterans Administration Medical Center and assistant professor of psychiatry at the Mount Sinai School of Medicine in New York City. He is an active investigator in family studies in AD as possible indicators of genetic causes. His present research centers on the degree to which the striking pattern of inheritance seen in familial AD may operate inconspicuously in other, more typical cases.

ROBERT N. BUTLER, M.D., is Brookdale Professor and chairman of the Gerald and May Ellen Ritter Department of Geriatrics and Adult Development, Mount Sinai Medical Center, New York City. He was the principal investigator of one of the first comprehensive longitudinal studies of the health of the elderly, conducted by the National Institute of Mental Health (1955–66), and was founding director of the National Institute on Aging (1975–82). In 1976, he won the Pulitzer Prize in nonfiction for *Why Survive? Being Old in America*. Dr. Butler is editor-in-chief of *Geriatrics*. He is a member of the Advisory Council of the New York–New Jersey Center on Environmental and Occupational Health, chairs programs for the Commonwealth and Brookdale foundations, serves on the Physician's Payment Review Commission of the U.S. Congress, and helped found the American Federation for Aging Research and the Alzheimer's Disease and Related Disorders Association, upon whose boards he serves.

DAVID F. CHAVKIN, J.D., is the directing attorney of the Maryland Disability Law Center, Maryland's protective and advocacy system for disabled children and adults. He is a former deputy director of the office of civil rights of the U.S. Department of Health and Human Services and former managing attorney of the National Health Law Program. He served as a consultant on the project on dementia of the U.S. Congressional Office of Technology Assessment.

HOWARD A. CRYSTAL, M.D., is assistant professor of neurology and codirector of neurogeriatrics at the Albert Einstein College of Medicine. He is currently researching clinicopathological correlates of AD and is conducting studies of biological markers and drug treatments.

PETER DAVIES, PH.D., is professor of pathology and neuroscience at the Albert Einstein College of Medicine. He is a member of the ADRDA Medical and Scientific Advisory Board and has received several awards for his research on AD, most recently the City of New York Liberty Medal in 1986 and the Metropolitan Life Foundation Award in 1987. His current research is focused on identifying a diagnostic indicator of AD in living patients.

NANCY N. DUBLER, LL.B., is the director of the division of legal and ethical issues in health care in the Department of Epidemiology and Social Medicine of the Montefiore Medical Center/Albert Einstein College of Medicine in New York City. She has written and lectured extensively on issues of geriatrics, gerontology, and law. She was coeditor of a book entitled *Alzheimer's Dementia: Dilemmas in Clinical Research.*

MICHAEL GILFIX, J.D., has devoted much of his legal career to the concerns of the elderly. His professional memberships include the medical ethics committee of El Camino Hospital in California and the estate-planning section of the State Bar of California. He has served as president of the Association of Legal Programs for Older Californians. Mr. Gilfix has lectured and written extensively on legal services for the elderly, as well as on the particular concerns of Alzheimer patients. He maintains his law offices in Palo Alto and San Francisco, California.

LISA P. GWYTHER, M.S.W., is an assistant professor and director of the Alzheimer's Family Support Program at the Duke University Center for the Study of Aging and Human Development in Durham, North Carolina. She is the author of the 1985 ADRDA publication *Care of Alzheimer's Patients: A Manual for Nursing Home Staff* and has published several articles on AD patients and their families.

LISSY F. JARVIK, M.D., PH.D., is professor of psychiatry at the University of California, Los Angeles, chief of neuropsychogeriatrics at UCLA's Neuropsychiatric Institute and Hospital, and chief of psychogeriatrics at the Brentwood Veterans Administration Medical Center. Dr. Jarvik's research has been concerned with human genetics, with mental functioning, with depression and dementia of the Alzheimer type, and with the effect of drugs. She has written over 200 articles, has edited a dozen volumes, is on numerous editorial boards, and is founding coeditor of the new

Alzheimer's Disease and Associated Disorders—An International Journal. In 1986, Dr. Jarvik received the Jack Weinberg Memorial Award for geriatric psychiatry from the American Psychiatric Association, the Robert W. Kleemeier Award for outstanding research in the field of aging from the Gerontological Society of America, and the Edward B. Allen Award for special contribution to the field of geriatric psychiatry from the American Geriatrics Society.

ROBERT KATZMAN, M.D., is the Florence Riford Professor for Research in Alzheimer's Disease and professor and chair of the department of neurosciences at the University of California, San Diego. He was the founding chairman of the Medical and Scientific Advisory Board of ADRDA from 1979 to 1985. In 1985, he was the first recipient of the Allied Achievement in Aging Award, and he received the American Geriatrics Society Henderson Memorial Award in 1986. He is past president of the American Neurological Association.

ROCHELLE LIPKOWITZ, R.N., M.S., is a psychiatric nurse-clinician at the Pride of Judea Mental Health Center in New York. She has been a consultant to the New York chapter of ADRDA and is co-leader of a support group for AD caregivers. She has lectured widely to health-care professionals and family members and has a special interest in risk factors in caregivers.

NANCY E. LOMBARDO, PH.D., is a vice-president of the national ADRDA and chairs its Chapter Committee. She has a Ph.D. in political science from Yale University and has evaluated federal health and manpower programs for several years. Her mother has had AD for over twenty years. Dr. Lombardo has lectured extensively on the disease at various professional association meetings.

JEAN MARKS, M.A., is the associate executive director of the New York chapter of ADRDA, where she is responsible for education and family services. She has spoken on behalf of the chapter to various community groups. She has a master's degree in psychological counseling from Columbia University. Ms. Marks's father had AD.

RENEE POLLACK, M.S.W., is the executive director of Westchester Community Services. She has been a member of several community organizations, including the Westchester County Board of Mental Health. She has served as president of the New York State chapter of the National Association of Social Workers and is currently chairperson of the Education Committee of the national ADRDA.

KATHRYN C. REES, M.A., is a legislative advocate and political consultant representing interests in the health-care arena, including the California chapters of ADRDA. She has represented public hospitals, children's hospitals, and the California Hospital Association, as well as myriad individual interests and health-care provider groups. Ms. Rees specializes in developing systems for effective grass-roots lobbying. She is a frequent lecturer on public affairs and California politics and serves on the executive committee of the Institute of Governmental Advocates.

MARION ROACH, a free-lance writer living in New York City, is the author of the book *Another Name for Madness*. As the daughter of an Alzheimer patient, she has lectured around the country on the problems of caregivers. She has testified before the New York State legislature and the U.S. Congress on the problems of family members of AD patients.

KATHLEEN WESTROPP STAUBER, PH.D., A.C.S.W., is a professor of social welfare and social work at Mundelein College in Chicago. She has a counseling and consultation practice with adolescents and their families. Dr. Stauber codeveloped and led the training program for lay leaders in the Second-Generation Program, a Chicago ADRDA support group for children and grandchildren of Alzheimer's disease patients. She is presently writing a book on family therapy, to be published in 1988.

PETER J. STRAUSS, J.D., is a partner in the firm of Strauss and Wolff, which devotes the major portion of its practice to legal counseling for the aged and their families in the areas of retirement planning, Medicaid, Medicare, Social Security disability, financial planning, and planning for catastrophic illness and physical and mental disability.

LEON J. THAL, M.D., is chief of neurology at the San Diego Veterans Administration Medical Center and associate professor of neurosciences at the University of California, San Diego. He also codirects a geropsychiatry evaluation and treatment unit at the San Diego VA Medical Center. His research is currently focused on the treatment of memory loss in AD.

DAVID W. TRADER, M.D., is a postdoctoral fellow in geriatric psychiatry in the Department of Biobehavioral Sciences at the University of California, Los Angeles. Dr. Trader's research activities include studies of psychopharmacologic treatments of multi-infarct dementia and Alzheimer's disease. He was an invitee to the National Institute of Mental Health workshop "Depression in Alzheimer's Disease: Component or Consequence?" held in June 1986.

JULIET WARSHAUER is one of the founders of the Westchester chapter of ADRDA and a past president of that chapter, after serving as vice-president for four years. The widow of an Alzheimer patient, she has participated in several radio and television programs on AD and has written an article on it for *The New York Times*.

MARCELLA BAKUR WEINER, ED.D., is an adjunct professor in the Department of Psychology at Brooklyn College of CUNY. She is a practicing psychotherapist in New York City and the author of numerous articles and several books dealing with aging.

ELAINE S. YATZKAN, A.C.S.W., is a clinical social worker with a special interest in aging and the families of the elderly. She is the social-work supervisor at the Resnick Gerontology Center of the Albert Einstein College of Medicine in New York. Mrs. Yatzkan is a founding member and on the board of directors of the New York chapter of ADRDA. Mrs. Yatzkan is an author of several articles regarding AD.

Index

371

About the Editor

MIRIAM K. ARONSON, ED.D., a social gerontologist, is associate professor of neurology and psychiatry at the Albert Einstein College of Medicine in New York City. She has long-standing interests in the psychosocial aspects of aging, the development and impact of dementing illness, and the development and implementation of long-term-care services and policies, and has been involved in research, service, and teaching. She is the principal investigator of a ten-year longitudinal study of the development of dementia in "old-old" persons.

Dr. Aronson is publications editor of Alzheimer's Disease and Related Disorders Association (ADRDA) and education consultant to this national organization. She was editor of the *Newsletter* for seven years and a member of the New York State Board of Nursing Home Examiners for six years. She is a member of the public policy committee and the executive committee of the Social Research, Planning and Policy Section of the Gerontological Society of America; of the program committee of the American Orthopsychiatric Association; of the New York State Board of Nursing Home Examiners; and of the Mayor's (New York City) Advisory Board on Alzheimer's Disease. Dr. Aronson has given more than 150 presentations nationally and internationally and has a growing list of publications.